Clinical Information Systems in Critical Care

Cecily Morrison

Researcher in Health and Information Systems
University of Cambridge, UK

Matthew R. Jones

University Lecturer in Information Systems
Judge Business School
University of Cambridge, UK

Julie Bracken

Critical Care Matron
Papworth Hospital
Cambridge, UK

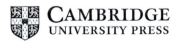

CAMBRIDGE
UNIVERSITY PRESS

CAMBRIDGE
UNIVERSITY PRESS

University Printing House, Cambridge CB2 8BS, United Kingdom

Published in the United States of America by Cambridge University Press,
New York

Cambridge University Press is part of the University of Cambridge.

It furthers the University's mission by disseminating knowledge in the pursuit of
education, learning and research at the highest international levels of excellence.

www.cambridge.org
Information on this title: www.cambridge.org/9780521156745

© Cecily Morrison, Matthew R. Jones and Julie Bracken 2014

First published 2014

Printed in the United Kingdom by CPI Group Ltd, Croydon CR0 4YY

A catalogue record for this publication is available from the British Library

Library of Congress Cataloguing in Publication data
Morrison, Cecily, author.
Clinical information systems in critical care / Cecily Morrison, Matthew R. Jones,
Julie Bracken.
   p.   ;   cm. – (Core critical care)
Includes bibliographical references and index.
ISBN 978-0-521-15674-5 (paperback)
I. Jones, Matthew R. (Matthew Russell), 1958– author.   II. Bracken, Julie, author.
III. Title.   IV. Series: Core critical care.
[DNLM: 1. Critical Care.   2. Health Information Systems.   WX 218]
RC86.7
616.02′80285 – dc23   2013026159

ISBN 978-0-521-15674-5 Paperback

Clinical Information Systems in Critical Care

CORE CRITICAL CARE

Series Editor

Dr Alain Vuylsteke

Papworth Hospital

Cambridge, UK

Assistant Editor

Jo-anne Fowles

Papworth Hospital

Cambridge, UK

Other titles in the series

Delirium in Critical Care

Valerie Page and E. Wesley Ely

ISBN 9780521132534

Intra-Abdominal Hypertension

Manu Malbrain and Jan De Waele

ISBN 9780521149396

Forthcoming titles in the series

Renal Replacement Therapy in Critical Care

Patrick Honoré and Oliver Joannes-Boyau

ISBN 9780521145404

CONTENTS

FOREWORD

Using a computer-based clinical information system (CIS) is, as the late informatics pioneer Homer Warner noted, 80% sociology and 20% technology. Today, the growth in use of these systems as well as their ever-widening applications have convinced me that clinicians who live 'for things to get back to normal' should just get over it since this isn't likely to happen any time soon. Instead, health information and communications technology keeps developing alongside an exponential growth in the science base of the healing professions as genomics is augmented by burgeoning chronic illness calling for 'activated' patients if good outcomes are to be expected. For those clinicians who are originators or early adopters, they're truly blessed to live in such compelling times, while for those clinicians who are either pragmatists or conservers, it can seem well beyond disruptive. It is hardly any wonder then, that the American Board of Medical Specialties recently added a Clinical Informatics certificate to its list of specialties and that chief clinical information officers are becoming the norm in larger US hospitals. Their roles are to assure that these systems can address those issues raised in the latter chapters of this volume.

As Sir Cyril Chantler noted, 'Medicine used to be simple, ineffective, and relatively safe. Now it is complex, effective and potentially dangerous.' When one is choosing and implementing clinical information systems for 24/7 critical care units characterized by complex life support equipment and decidedly constrained 'time windows' for critical decision-making, one needs reasoned and seasoned advice. This concise volume serves that purpose well.

In short, Morrison, Jones and Bracken did us all a favour by clearly laying out the most critical facets of this challenge whether one is a happy volunteer or the most reluctant conscript. Implementing clinical information systems has been described accurately as a 'contact sport'. The descriptions of relevant issues in the initial chapters are clear, honest, candid, and carry the message of experienced users that these systems are both 'works in progress' and genuine challenges but with much to offer to those willing to make the personal and financial investment. Despite the utility of CIS some issues remain with a stubborn consistency, including interoperability, clunky user-interfaces and system security. Yet training can make a difference. Convincing clinicians to undertake three or more hours of training can offset weeks of complaints from those who limit themselves to one hour.

The well-written section on documentation deserves particular commendation since often this effort is seen as somehow redundant. Since the focus is on critical care, patient engagement through CISs gets little attention. With the rise of chronic illness in aging populations, connectivity with patients to manage their care becomes a key factor for future success, for example adding the patient and perhaps even a key loved one to the 'clinical team'. Also, relating to governance may become a significant part of the business case negotiations and may prove to be problematic if taken for granted in some settings.

The reader will want to keep this handy guide available for ongoing reference since it is filled with hard earned wisdom. My compliments go to the authors for contributing a very useful addition to the clinical informatics literature. And my hopes and best wishes go to those who undertake the clinical transformation that CIS involves. Remember to celebrate your successes along the way; you've earned them.

Don Eugene Detmer, MD, MA
University of Virginia

Chapter 1

Introduction

What is a clinical information system?

Critical care is full of digital technology. Infusion pumps are automated, ventilators have digital interfaces to manage their functions, images are stored in a database, and administrative teams use information systems.

A clinical information system, referred to throughout this book as a CIS, is a piece of technology that supports the entire clinical process at the bedside.

A CIS provides the technology for the clinician to manage patient data and coordinate care. Its primary function is to compute, store and display data from various sources (Figure 1.1).

For example, it can store arterial blood gas results, compute fluid balance, and display heart rate over time. It structures data in the database, which makes it easier to retrieve historical data or collate a particular result across a cohort of patients.

A CIS also functions as a tool to coordinate patient care. It provides mechanisms to prescribe drugs, order investigations, communicate with healthcare professionals from all disciplines and document all patient care.

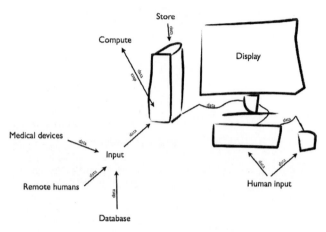

Figure 1.1 The clinical information system (CIS).

A CIS can be a tool that supports all aspects of patient care on a critical care unit (CCU).

CIS versus paper

A major difference between CISs and paper is the way that data can be integrated and viewed and used in patient care (Figure 1.2).

A CIS can provide a three-dimensional view of the data, with a bit of effort to overcome the two-dimensionality of the screen. It is easy to scroll backwards and forwards in time, viewing historical as well as current data. It is possible to juxtapose data, such as graphing blood pressure against heart rate one above the other (Figure 1.3).

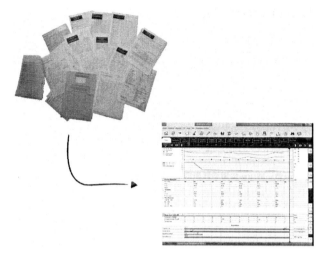

Figure 1.2 CIS: Transformation from paper to screen allows wider integration and organization. All data are contained in one location but can be accessed from many. Data can be organized (again and again) in many different ways.

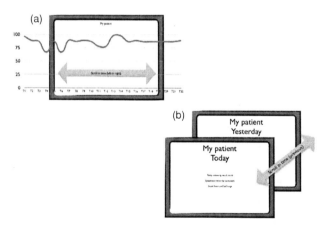

Figure 1.3 (a) Three-dimensional view of data: scrolling back in time, juxtaposing data from various sources, reviewing historical data. (b) Granularity of data: zooming in/out, e.g. reviewing time-point or trends over a long period.

Unlike paper, it is possible to alter the granularity of the data, zooming in to view particular data points and zooming out to view trends.

Introducing a CIS is a greater financial undertaking than developing paper forms. Yet it can also provide new ways of supporting care.

A CIS provides a more reliable tool to plan patient care, increasing legibility, consistency and accountability (Figure 1.4). As will be discussed in later chapters, this has advantages and disadvantages.

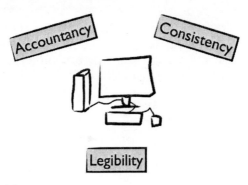

Figure 1.4

The formalization of work practices can cause problems, and the flexibility of paper in supporting communication can be missed. These problems can be overcome to reap the benefits of a CIS in most contexts.

CIS in different flavours

There are various CISs available, with many specialized for use in critical care.

The systems all have similar functions, but have differences that can be significant for the choices an institution makes.

Some systems support all aspects of patient care within the institution, while others are specific to the location (critical care being one) or task (be it administrative or clinical). Examples include some CISs encompassing all episodes from booking to theatre set-up, administration and payment. Others are specific to documentation and drug prescribing.

Not only do systems differ, but institutions may choose to use them in differing ways. Some prefer to maintain paper documentation, but interact with the pathology and pharmacy departments through an information system. Other CISs offer advanced features around clinical decision support, such as recommendations or alerts. The choice of utilization will depend on the requirements of the institution.

A significant difference between CISs is whether they are standard, customizable, or even customized by healthcare professionals. This changes dramatically how a CIS might be used and developed within an institution (Table 1.1).

Decisions

The range of available systems and possible applications underscores the number of decisions that need to be made when planning to introduce a CIS.

It is not possible to justify buying a CIS, or even to base a decision to buy one, entirely on proven benefit. As will be discussed throughout this book, benefits are specific to the suitability of a CIS to an institution and the way in which it is implemented.

Table 1.1 CIS and customization

Out of the box	The vendor sells a fully operational system – with no or little room for adaptation by the user.
Customizable	The vendor sells a system that can be tailored to some extent to the users' needs through interaction with a technical team (sometimes provided by the vendor).
User-customizable	The vendor sells the tools and training to allow the user to develop and maintain a custom-made system. The clinical team can customize the system.
Self-made	The system is made in-house by a team of enthusiastic medical computer experts. The clinical team is dependent on local expertise.

There may be many conflicting demands that will need to be resolved in choosing and implementing the CIS. For example, management might see the opportunity to collect data, but staff might resent having to spend an extra 30 minutes typing in data that they do not use. There may be other issues that arise between actual work practices and ideal work practices. The choice and implementation of a CIS requires careful consideration of the differing demands within the institution and realistic decision-making (Figure 1.5).

This book

This book discusses the issues that need to be considered when selecting and implementing a CIS in critical care. Common mistakes and pitfalls are highlighted. When appropriate, evidence is offered from research in health informatics and organizational change.

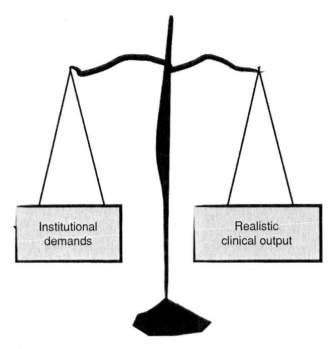

Figure 1.5

The authors and editors are healthcare professionals and university researchers who were all involved in the full implementation of a CIS in a large critical care unit.

The healthcare professionals bring their experience of leading the selection and implementation; the researchers add their knowledge from the research literature and the experience gained from observing and reflecting upon an implementation. These two viewpoints give this book a rich perspective from which to offer suggestions and guidance.

This book will not choose a system for the reader. The authors are not aware of specifics that will affect choices in a particular unit at various stages. They cannot resolve tensions in the institution that will result from the process of acquiring a CIS, such as differences in requirements and expectations of managers and clinicians.

This book is for all those involved in the selection, purchase, implementation and use of a CIS. This includes clinicians, nurses, allied healthcare professionals, managers and executives. It is key to the success of a CIS implementation project to include as many stakeholders as possible. This book can inform and support discussion between multiple stakeholders.

We hope this book will provide a useful guide to what may seem an opaque and risky process.

Chapter 2

Deciding to purchase a CIS

Introduction

Investing in a CIS will affect the operation of a critical care unit in many ways. Adjustments will need to be made to the budget, and staff will need to change the way they work.

To justify such significant changes, it is necessary to establish a coherent case. This chapter describes the key stages that are likely to be involved in developing such a case: review of the clinical vision, review of critical care unit capabilities and priorities, and learning from others' experience.

The need for a clinical vision

It is undisputed that a CIS needs to deliver clinical benefits to be considered useful and successful. To do so, a CIS must support the clinical vision of the unit.

An important stage in considering whether a CIS is suitable for a unit is to articulate how it fits with its clinical vision.

When embarking on a CIS purchase, the critical care unit clinical vision should be reviewed, or one should be established if none exists.

Table 2.1 Elements to review when defining the unit clinical vision

Commonly shared ideas about how clinical care can best be delivered
Knowledge of best practice from other comparable units
Specific problems with current delivery that need to be addressed
Specific interests of influential unit staff

The typical elements contributing to the development of the clinical vision are listed in Table 2.1.

The articulation of the clinical vision should encompass the views of all involved in the unit at any level and from a range of disciplines. This should lead to a concise statement of the vision that can serve as a reference point for the subsequent selection and implementation of the CIS.

This statement and its development can be an opportunity for collective reflection on the future direction of patient care in the unit and can help build a consensus.

The clinical vision should remain flexible. Those involved should be reminded that it is expected to evolve over time.

Time spent outside the clinical environment, such as during an away-day for selected staff, may help to foment the vision.

It is best to develop the clinical vision independently of CIS choice to avoid the temptation of developing a vision that matches the expected capabilities of the CIS. That is not to say that there may not be some iteration between the clinical vision and expected CIS capabilities. Considering how a CIS could contribute to clinical care may identify new

Table 2.2 Points to include in a review of the capabilities and priorities of the unit

---

1. Individual leadership capabilities
2. Project team capabilities
3. Staff attitudes
4. Staff competencies
5. Organizational competencies
6. Managerial attitudes and priorities
7. Health system priorities

---

opportunities to improve patient care, but the clinical vision should not deliberately be distorted to support the case for a CIS.

Poor compatibility between the clinical vision and the expected capabilities of a CIS should raise an alarm about whether a CIS is appropriate for the unit. This is especially true if the decision-makers are assuming that the CIS will perform as initially expected, which is unlikely.

Review of unit capabilities and priorities

The second step in deciding whether a CIS is an appropriate choice is to conduct a review to help identify the characteristics that may support or impede CIS introduction. Such a review should include the points listed in Table 2.2.

Understanding of the key points in relation to each of these characteristics within the unit will help identify areas of vulnerability before the project begins.

Individual leadership capabilities

Research into CIS implementations unequivocally indicates that successful adoption requires strong leadership within the unit.

Although leadership may be shared among a team, there is usually one individual, often called the CIS Champion, who is recognized as the chief proponent and architect of the CIS. If the CIS is to achieve clinical acceptance it is recognized that this individual should be a senior clinician, preferably the Unit Director.

Ask yourself early in the process if you have someone who could fulfil that role.

The effectiveness of the CIS Champion is not simply a product of their title, but will depend on the quality of their leadership and their circumstances. It is essential that the Champion is able to engage and lead a strong team to deliver the project. The task of implementing a CIS will be beyond the capabilities of a single individual.

The Champion's leadership will need to extend beyond the project team to motivate and manage unit staff before, during and after CIS implementation. As this time span is normally about three years, the Champion role is a long-term commitment which is difficult to hand over to another individual. Ideally the CIS Champion is a staff member expected to stay in the same senior post for at least three years.

The literature on change management identifies three types of leadership situation that may be favourable for the initiation

Table 2.3 Favourable leadership situations

1. Established leader anticipating environmental pressures for change
   Achieving change is likely to be easier when there is a plausible external
   pressure to which the CIS provides a response. This pressure may be
   budgetary, regulatory, due to changing work practices, or a new technology.
   The external nature of the pressure motivates people to change as the unit has
   little control over the situation. It allows adequate planning as the changes are
   anticipated.
2. Established leader with strong personal support
   Change does not necessarily require external threat. It may be initiated by an
   established leader in whose vision unit staff have confidence. Such change
   may be highly dependent on the personal qualities of the individual and may
   face problems when they are no longer around to maintain it.
3. New leader
   A change in leadership can often be a catalyst for new initiatives, both as the new
   leader seeks to demonstrate their distinctiveness, and because they may enjoy
   a 'honeymoon period' in which criticism of their vision and abilities is relaxed.

of a project involving significant organizational change such as
a CIS implementation (Table 2.3).

Project team capabilities

A CIS implementation cannot be done by one person.
Successful implementation requires a project team.

Before deciding to start on the project it is a good idea to
consider whether the necessary competencies are available to
staff the project team.

The team should have people with a variety of skills and
strengths: some who are good at articulating the vision and
communicating it to others, and others who are better at detail

and checking that things are done correctly. The team should include people who have some information technology (IT) and project management skills. These may be primarily supplied externally (for example by the CIS vendor) but it is beneficial to have in-house people on the team with experience of similar projects.

The project team should include individuals from different stakeholder groups to ensure that all views are represented. While some of the team responsibilities may reflect professional roles, it is valuable to cast the net widely and to recruit able individuals even if the skills they bring are not part of their usual role.

When selecting a project team, it is advisable to plan, where possible, both the duration that team members are likely to remain in post (and therefore able to continue in this role) and whether commitments of their existing role are likely to restrict their future contribution.

Investment in the project team is high in term of time and training, and inability to carry this forward can prove costly.

It is very costly to devote considerable time to training a senior member of staff and later find out that clinical and managerial demands mean it is impossible for such a person to fulfil the expected role.

Staff attitudes

Staff acceptance of a CIS is crucial to its success.

It is important to gauge staff attitudes towards the project. Staff members who have positive views about change, and about introduction of a CIS more specifically, may naturally gravitate towards the project team. This can give a distorted picture of staff attitudes as a whole.

It is necessary to take careful account of the variety and distribution of attitudes and to make efforts to 'sound out' the views of those who may have negative attitudes towards change and CIS. Although it is important not to typecast individuals, it can be helpful to identify whether negative attitudes are more prevalent among particular groups of staff. For example, some senior clinicians may be concerned about their work being subject to greater control, or about their lack of computer skills creating a poor impression.

Negative attitudes towards change and the CIS should not be dismissed as unreasonable 'resistance', as these may reflect personal experience of previous failed change initiatives or scepticism towards claims that information technology (IT) can transform healthcare.

Understanding concerns and assessing actions to address them can alleviate some negative perceptions. The project team as a whole needs to be sensitive to these resistors, and understand that fear and uncertainty may underlay their attitude.

The team needs to ensure that they do not take negative comments personally; effective support and debriefing opportunities within the project team itself will help members maintain a balanced outlook.

Establishing a support network becomes even more important as the implementation date approaches.

Staff competencies

Using a CIS will necessarily involve use of a computer, so a major issue in deciding whether to adopt a CIS will be the computer literacy of staff.

It may be that some staff already have experience of computer use in aspects of their work or may be keen users of information technology outside work. For those who lack computing skills the prospect of using a CIS may be a source of considerable stress that may affect their work. Identifying these individuals and developing plans to support them in overcoming their anxieties is necessary to avoid later difficulties.

Staff competencies can be formally assessed. One way to do this is through a simple survey or an activity.

One critical care unit created a simple exercise to click on buttons on the screen with a mouse to establish the computer literacy levels of their staff and determine what specific issues might need addressing. Not only was this revealing about staff computer competency, it helped build confidence among those staff with less or no IT experience (Figure 2.1).

Assumptions should never be made about the level of IT competence. Although computers form a large part of daily life these days, there are still significant numbers of staff (from all disciplines) who do not have basic IT skills.

Organizational competencies

The work involved in implementing a CIS will not be restricted to the critical care unit, so the competencies of the wider

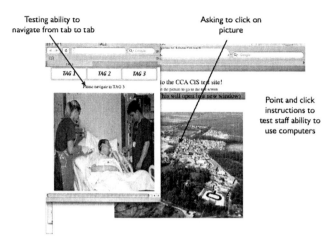

Figure 2.1 Never make assumptions about the level of IT knowledge within your workforce.

hospital are likely to be a significant factor in the project's success.

A critical care unit in a hospital that is open to innovation, and more specifically IT, is likely to face fewer difficulties than one in a hospital that is very set in its ways and has low levels of IT use.

Relationships with other departments are important. Departments that interact directly with the critical care unit in ways that the CIS may alter are likely to be affected, as well as those that may feel threatened by developments in critical care, either in terms of competition to innovate or concerns at the resources and management attention that the CIS may divert.

It is important to consider other departments from the initial stages and engage them early on to minimize objections when implementation starts. It might be useful to draw interdependency charts at an early stage to understand who will be affected (Figure 2.2).

One unit's experience showed that the greatest resistance, once the system was in place, came from the clinical areas outside of critical care. This is often difficult to judge in the planning stages as an 'ostrich' approach often accompanies any discussion on potential impacts.

The department most affected by the introduction of a CIS is often the hospital IT department. CIS success will, to some extent, rely on the cooperation of the IT department.

Although some IT departments may welcome clinical leadership in adopting a CIS, others may feel threatened by it. Some IT departments may have experience of CISs, or similar systems, elsewhere in the hospital and may be a source of expert advice. For others, it may be a new venture in which they are learning as much as the critical care unit.

Although clinicians and IT staff often approach problems in different ways, it pays to make the effort to work together, as a good relationship will substantially ease the process of solving problems that will undoubtedly arise once the CIS is implemented.

Resources within an IT department need to be considered as the CIS will increase demands on the department, not just at the planning and implementation stage, but ongoing.

Issues such as 24 hour cover in case of system failure need to be addressed before implementation.

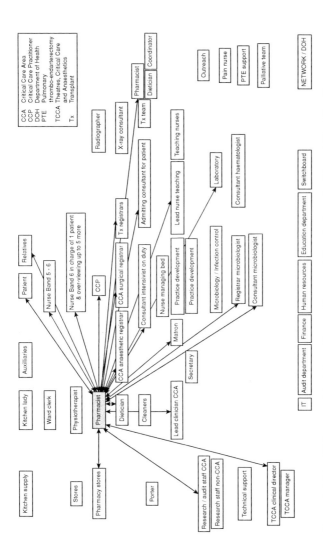

CCA   Critical Care Area
CCP   Critical Care Practitioner
DOH   Department of Health
PTE   Pulmonary
       thrombo-endarterectomy
TCCA   Theatres, Critical Care
       and Anaesthetics
Tx   Transplant

Kitchen supply

Stores

Pharmacy stores

Porter

Research / audit staff CCA
Research staff non-CCA

Technical support

TCCA clinical director
TCCA manager

Kitchen lady
Ward clerk

Physiotherapist

Pharmacist

Dietician

Cleaners

Lead clinician CCA

Secretary

Auxiliaries

Patient
Nurse Band 5 - 6

Nurse Band 6 in charge of 1 patient
& over-viewing up to 5 more

CCP

CCA anaesthetic registrar
CCA surgical registrar
Consultant intensivist on duty

Nurse managing bed

Matron

Practice development
Practice development

Microbiology / Infection control

Registrar microbiologist
Consultant microbiologist

Relatives

Tx registrars

Admitting consultant for patient

Lead nurse teaching

Laboratory

Consultant haematologist

Radiographer

X-ray consultant

Tx team
Pharmacist
Dietician Coordinator

Teaching nurses

Outreach

Pain nurse

PTE support

Palliative team

IT   Audit department   Finance   Human resources   Education department   Switchboard   NETWORK / DOH

Figure 2.2 Identifying people's interactions will support the design of a CIS and identify all stakeholders.

Managerial attitudes and priorities

Another significant influence on CIS implementation is the attitudes and competencies of the institutional management.

A management team that has little knowledge of, or interest in, IT may provide little support for the introduction of a CIS or they may be happy to be guided by clinical interests if a convincing argument can be made.

Understanding the priorities and interests of management may be valuable both in deciding whether to purchase a CIS and in preparing the case for a CIS (see Chapter 3).

It is important to understand the decision-making and procurement processes within the institution. Understanding these processes will identify those to whom the case for adopting a CIS will need to be made, and the steps to be followed if the case is approved.

Health system priorities

Attitudes and priorities within an institution will generally be shaped by those within the broader health system.

If a CIS can be shown to be aligned with national priorities, for example, this is likely to favour its adoption. If national attitudes are shaped by negative experiences in other settings or if funding is restricted, then it is likely to be more difficult to gain support for implementing a CIS.

News stories about IT failures in national initiatives such as the UK NHS National Programme for IT (NPfIT) may make the CIS case more difficult to argue.

Learning from others' experience

Carrying out such a preliminary review of the unit may be difficult if project team members have had little prior experience of information system implementation, or of large project investments.

It may be particularly valuable for team members to gain insight on the benefits and pitfalls of adopting a CIS through visits and discussions with sites that have already been through the process.

Direct observation of how a CIS works in practice in different institutions is recognized as one of the most effective ways of assessing how well a CIS is likely to translate to a local setting. This is an opportunity to discover the lessons that others have learned that will help implementation run more smoothly.

While it is helpful to visit units with a similar clinical focus, it is equally valuable to visit units that deal with very different groups of patients.

For example, a cardiothoracic critical care unit and a burns unit have differing average length of stay and therefore use their CIS in dissimilar ways. Crossing such boundaries can spur ideas about new ways of working or help to surface 'taken-for-granted' assumptions about care practices that may be challenged by CIS adoption.

It is valuable for these visits to involve staff in different roles and not be restricted to enthusiasts for the CIS. A diverse team offers a broader perspective on how a system may fit into unit practices and how these practices might change.

Including people with negative attitudes towards CIS will help to allay concerns by providing them with an opportunity to see a system in action. They may also ask important, if awkward, questions that enthusiasts could overlook.

Asking to meet a cross-section of staff rather than just the CIS administrator or lead implementor will be valuable. Speaking to the end users will highlight many previously unthought-of ideas, and contact with the training team can give a better understanding of challenges ahead.

Such visits help build a strong foundation on which to make decisions about which CIS to buy and how to implement it. They can introduce greater realism about the work involved, inform planning and help build a team who are confident, fully engaged and ready to support implementation.

Reports from international exemplar sites such as Regenstrief Institute, Brigham and Women's Hospital or Veterans National may be persuasive in supporting the case for CIS investment.

Table 2.4 Key questions before purchasing a CIS

Key questions	Why?
Is there a strong, credible clinical lead?	Essential for driving forward the project and engaging colleagues
Is there a clear up-to-date clinical vision?	Can be used to support the business case for introduction of a CIS
Do available CISs fit with the clinical vision?	If it is not possible to fit the two together, a CIS may not be right for the unit.
Are you able to build a strong and effective project team?	Success of the project will rest largely on the project team.
Are staff attitudes supportive to a CIS (or at least not wholly negative)?	Support from key staff outside of the project team will positively affect all staff members.
Have you considered the impact on other departments within the hospital?	Awareness of impact on other areas and demands allows for more effective planning.
Have you managerial support (and if so, why)?	Strong managerial support will be key to success but be aware of the reasons for this support – check they are realistic.
Have you seen the system working elsewhere?	There is no substitute for seeing the system in a clinical setting and understanding what it can and cannot do.

Key questions to ask before embarking on a CIS purchase

Table 2.4 summarizes some of the key questions to be considered before deciding to invest in a CIS.

These questions do not presume that the answers will necessarily support CIS adoption. If there are serious concerns at any level, it may be necessary to review whether these can be resolved or whether they are sufficient to jeopardize the success of the project.

Key point

- A decision to purchase a CIS suggests that the CIS supports the clinical vision, that the critical care unit has the right capabilities and priorities, and that efforts have been made to learn about the advantages and disadvantages of a CIS through visits to other units.

Chapter 3

Making the case

Introduction

This chapter discusses how a business case can be made for a CIS.

It begins with a discussion of how to determine the cost and benefits of a CIS and then suggests how these might be collated into a business case.

Costs and benefits

The decision to buy a CIS ultimately rests on the benefits being greater than the costs. A preparatory step then is to balance benefits against costs.

This can be a tricky process as hidden costs need to be accounted for and the benefits can be difficult to quantify.

This section lists the common costs, discusses the benefits that can result from using a CIS, and provides some cautionary advice on presenting them accurately in a business plan.

Costs

Direct expenditure associated with the purchase and implementation of a CIS, such as those involved in buying the software and hardware required to operate the system, are relatively easy to identify.

These direct expenditures are only a small part of the total cost. It is estimated that the five-year cost of ownership for major computing systems can be five to eight times the hardware and software acquisition costs.

Other common and easily recognized costs relate to installation and maintenance. These include the purchase and installation of necessary cabling and any other infrastructure required, including carts and wireless routers, as well as recurrent costs such as software licences and hardware and software maintenance.

Allowance may need to be made for upgrade and replacement of hardware and software over the lifetime of the project.

Staffing costs will be associated with CIS implementation to account for necessary activities, such as training and customization.

Training costs should include the cost of the trainers and training facilities and the staff time required to undertake the training.

It is important to consider the time it will take to train new recruits (arriving after the CIS implementation) and top-up training as aspects of the system change.

Experience has shown that new staff need much less training in terms of time than the staff present when a system is implemented. This is probably because they do not have to 'unlearn' and then 'relearn' a new system and are not hampered by existing ideas. Nevertheless, training for new staff still has to be factored into planning, and CIS training will need to be included in all new staff members' induction.

Another substantial cost is project management. CIS implementation is a large project and needs to be managed. This may be done professionally by an information systems project manager, by an in-house secondment, or by existing staff. In all these cases, funds will need to be allocated for the time spent on project management.

Utilizing 'in-house' staff to manage the project does not avoid costs as staff resources will have to be devoted to overseeing project implementation. If no project manager is employed, this task is likely to fall to senior critical care staff whose skills in this domain may be untested and the opportunity costs of whose diversion to CIS project management may be significant (even if unaccounted for).

There may be a variety of other, less-evident but potentially unavoidable, costs. One such cost that may have a significant influence on the effectiveness of a CIS in critical care settings is its integration with devices and information systems already in place. The costs of an interface to enable the CIS to access data will depend on the particular devices and systems installed, some of which may prove impossible to integrate with, or perhaps may only be integrated by incurring additional costs to upgrade legacy systems.

Integration may be dependent on third-party suppliers or internal departments over which the CIS project may have limited impact. Integration costs may be difficult to estimate in advance and are highly dependent on the particular setting in which the system is to be operated.

There may be similar uncertainty and unpredictability with staff-related costs. It may be expected, for example, that productivity will decrease while staff are trained to use the CIS. In some settings this may be considered a short-term effect. In settings with high levels of staff turnover, it may be a persistent issue.

There may be costs associated with ongoing user support and development and training related to system changes and upgrades.

It is better to err on the side of caution and overestimate integration costs and staff-related expenses.

Table 3.1 summarizes the main cost items associated with the implementation of a CIS.

Benefits

Benefits from a CIS are multiple, but they are often difficult to predict and measure.

Some claims rely on assumptions that the CIS will actually deliver efficiency improvements, which may not always be the case (at least to the extent expected).

Such assumptions include expected staff savings through speeding up of work practices, improved efficiency and elimination of redundant tasks (such as processing paper records) and the costs associated with paper record purchase, use and storage.

Table 3.1 Main cost items

Category	Cost item
Direct initial purchase costs	Hardware purchase
	Infrastructure
	Software purchase and/or licences
	Interfaces to devices and systems
Indirect initial purchase costs	Replacement/upgrade of equipment to interface with CIS
Direct recurrent costs	Hardware maintenance and upgrade
	Software maintenance and upgrade
	Consumables
Direct initial staff costs	Training – costs of trainers and training facilities
	Training – costs of staff time
	Customization
	Project management
Direct recurrent staff costs	User support
	Ongoing training
	Ongoing customization
Indirect staff costs	Loss of productivity during training
	Management time
	Possible resistance / loss of morale among staff

Reductions in staff turnover due to improved work practices may be predicted.

A CIS often means that work practices change, staff do different things and perhaps more safely or conveniently, but this may not necessarily improve efficiency.

One frequently predicted benefit of a CIS is time savings, as staff no longer have to calculate results by hand or search for paper records, and data is immediately communicated to relevant parties. A consistent research finding, however, is that time savings from CIS are rarely realized. Time 'saved' is used for other activities, which may take longer, such as keyboard entry of data.

It is wise to highlight how the CIS meets a clinical vision and avoid predicting tangible outcomes, particularly efficiency-related ones.

Another benefit from a CIS may be a by-product of the collation and integration of easily searchable data. This will be most useful for research and audit (although the direct benefits of this may be hard to quantify), but may enable managers to achieve savings through the better understanding of expenditure patterns. It may not be possible to estimate in advance the benefits achievable from such measures, as the opportunities will only be apparent once the system is in place.

Other benefits of a CIS are more difficult to quantify and include effects on staff morale, on staff attitudes towards changes in work practices, or on the particular critical care unit's reputation within its hospital or even within the wider critical care community.

Benefits that may not be directly attributable to the CIS, such as improvements in the quality of patient care, may arise.

Unfortunately, causality is often complex and the specific contribution of the CIS may be difficult to isolate. The 'Hawthorne effect' suggests that improvements in quality of care (or, equally, staff morale) could reflect the greater attention paid to staff during CIS implementation rather than the technology itself.

It is important to be cautious about which benefits are attributed to the CIS so that unreasonable expectations are not set up that will lead to the system being seen as a failure if they are not met.

Further benefits may only be apparent once a system is established. A drop in morale often accompanies initial implementation, owing to factors such as fear, uncertainty and the need for a steep learning curve. It is important to acknowledge this when considering the timeframe in which the business case intends to realize benefits.

Reduction of medication errors is a case in point when considering benefits from a CIS. CIS leads to a reduction of medication errors, owing to improved legibility of records, error-trapping checks, and alerts to warn clinicians of interactions. While there is a substantial literature supporting this case, it is also shown that CIS may introduce new types of error and that reductions may not be sustained (for example because clinicians pay progressively less attention to alerts over time). It may be risky to assume that such benefits will necessarily be sustainably achieved.

Box 3.1

One unit demonstrated a great reduction in medication errors sustained one year after introduction of the system. Over time, new systematic errors started to appear and were partly attributed to a new culture of 'click and go' rather than the expected 'click and check' by which the clinicians would ensure accuracy and ownership of any prescription. Some new systematic errors at the point of delivery were the results of minute differences in screen configuration that led to recurrent problems.

Table 3.2 Main benefits

Category	Benefit
Direct cash-releasing benefits	Elimination of redundant tasks
	Improved efficiency of tasks
	Elimination of costs associated with paper records
Indirect potential cash-releasing benefits	Better data for management of costs
Direct potential non-cash-releasing benefits	Time savings
	Reductions in medication errors
	Data for audit and research
Indirect non-cash-releasing benefits	Improved staff morale
	Unit reputation
	Changed staff attitudes

A CIS is likely to offer a number of tangible and intangible benefits as summarized in Table 3.2.

Cost-benefit analysis

The cost–benefit analysis is traditionally one of the bases for a business case that seeks to attribute benefits to the implementation of a CIS that significantly outweigh its costs.

When cost–benefit analysis is conducted for use in the business case, it can provide an incentive for underestimation of outlays and optimism in the calculation of the returns to be obtained from the system.

A realistic appraisal of costs and benefits will avoid later problems of unanticipated cost-overruns and unrealized benefits. Estimating costs and benefits is not straightforward; ask other units that have CIS about the costs and benefits associated with their system when visiting during the exploration stage.

Box 3.2

One unit recent research paper investigated an overspend of 35% (approximately $1 million) on a CIS implementation in three critical care units.

They found that: software costs were 7% more than budgeted; hardware costs were 8% more than budgeted; and personnel costs were 139% higher than anticipated. Personnel accounted for 83% of the underestimated costs.

Their findings give warning of the substantial amount of personnel time that is needed and therefore needs to be budgeted.

The business case

The previous section laid the groundwork for making the business case for a CIS.

Although a business case can sometimes be regarded as a 'convenient fiction' to meet the requirements of organizational budgeting procedures, it can have real consequences for a CIS project.

It sets performance and outcome expectations that may subsequently be used as measures of success and establishes benefit targets that may be 'realized' whether or not the system has actually achieved them.

It is therefore worth investing effort to ensure that the case is realistic in terms of costs, timescales and outcomes. The actual process of preparing the case may be of value by providing an

Table 3.3 A business case – four broad areas

1. Strategic fit	How does the scope of the proposed project fit within the existing business and IT/estate strategies (where relevant) of the organization?
	Is there a compelling case for change, when considering the existing and future operational needs of the organization?
2. Options appraisal	Document the different options that have been considered for addressing the organization's existing and future business needs.
	Aim to arrive at the optimum balance of cost, benefit and risk.
3. Affordability	Provide a broad estimate of the expected cost of the project over its whole lifetime.
	It may include options for financing the project.
4. Achievability	Set out the project organization and actions which will be undertaken to support the achievement of intended outcomes.

opportunity for a thorough and systematic assessment of expectations regarding the CIS.

A business case should normally address four broad areas shown in Table 3.3.

Each institution is likely to have its own business case format that will need to be followed, but it can be helpful to gather examples of business cases from other centres to see how these are organized and the categories addressed.

Other ideas may be gained from example business cases of CIS suppliers, but these must be used carefully as they are likely to be written to favour a particular system.

The headings of a standard business case are shown in Table 3.4.

Table 3.4 Standard business case

Heading	Description
Background	Describes the problem or clinical vision and discusses how the CIS would be part of this potential change. Addresses why the CIS is needed now and what the implications are of not doing it.
Scope	Describes what the scope of the project is, its purpose, key objectives and deliverables.
Objectives	Summarizes what the project is expected to achieve when it has been completed. Objectives should normally be 'SMART': specific, measurable, achievable, realistic and timely.
Strategic fit	Describes how the project fits with organizational strategies.
Options	Describes and evaluates the different options and gives reasons why the preferred option was chosen.
Proposed Solution	Identifies the selected option and explains how change will be implemented.
Benefits	Summarizes the main benefits, who is responsible for them and how they will be realized. Where possible, benefits should be expressed in financial terms to allow them to be weighed against costs and so that alternative options can be systematically compared. Benefits that are not quantifiable should be identified to avoid them being overlooked.
Risks	Identifies the key risks impacting the project and how it is proposed to manage them.
Dependencies	Identifies events or work that are either dependent on the outcome of this project or that the project will depend on.
Affordability	Identifies the resources that will be required, including staff resources, and where these resources will come from. Those responsible for providing resources must indicate they have approved the undertaking.

(*cont.*)

Table 3.4 (*cont.*)

Heading	Description
Analysis of costs and phasing of expenditure	Analyses the costs and indicates the phasing of expenditures.
Change control procedures	Explains how a change of personnel, scope or objectives will be handled.
Critical success factors	Outlines what must go right to ensure the success of the project in delivering the objectives and benefits. Does the project need to deliver all objectives and benefits to be successful?

Key points

- Ensure that the business plan is realistic in balancing costs and benefits.
- A case for the CIS needs to be in place before a purchase is made.
- Development of a business case and selection are likely to happen in parallel.

TO LEARN MORE

Further information on general business cases can be found in many specific textbooks. Various organizations and Departments of Health of diverse countries have sample business cases available to download.

Harvard Business Review Press, 2010. *Developing a Business Case: Expert Solutions to Everyday Challenges* (Harvard Pocket Mentor Series), Boston, MA: Harvard Business School Press.

M. J. Schmidt, 2009. *Business Case Essentials: A Guide to Structure and Content*, 3rd edn. Boston, MA: Solution Matrix.

For a more healthcare-oriented guide:

NorthWest London CLAHRC, available at: www.clahrc-northwestlondon.nihr.ac.uk/inc/files/documents/cld-resources/writing_a_business_case_handbook.pdf

Chapter 4

Choosing a CIS

Introduction

Choosing a CIS requires understanding the links between software, hardware and other devices. Each of them is integrated in a bigger system. Some requirements can be mutually exclusive and it is sometimes necessary to make trade-offs.

Choosing the best user interface is paramount but one cannot choose the interface independently of the vendor and associated support network.

Making choices and trade-offs

Envisaging the ideal system

Before beginning to explore the possibilities of each system on offer and becoming overwhelmed by choice, it is necessary to imagine the ideal system in detail. Decision should then be based on this ideal solution.

This ideal solution should be linked with the clinical vision, as discussed in Chapter 2. The aim is to ensure that the CIS will support the clinical vision.

Table 4.1 Questions to ask when imagining the CIS in place

What does the CIS look like?

How are staff using it?

What are they doing?

What are they not doing?

Is there anything in this picture that looks awkward or unwieldy?

Once an idea has been established about the role of the CIS clinically, the ideal system can be specified concretely by thinking about what parts of the current (paper-based) system should be retained and which need to change. This exercise should not be restricted to what is already familiar from current systems, but should consider new opportunities.

In imagining the ideal system it is important to be realistic. As a simple exercise to test how realistic a vision is, imagine staff moving around the unit doing their tasks and answer the questions listed in Table 4.1.

This exercise can be repeated for a number of common scenarios, for example ward rounds, emergency interventions and bedside care.

If it is not possible to imagine staff using the system, it is unlikely that they will adapt to it.

As well as being realistic, it is important to be adventurous. Information systems will change the way that people think about data, and ultimately the way they work. Although this may be very difficult to imagine or predict in advance, it is a likelihood that is best planned for. Space should be left for the clinical vision to adapt as the CIS allows the unit to work in different ways.

This is important for systems that are to be in place for a substantial time, for example ten years, as one can expect the development of the clinical environment to be substantial in that period.

It is unlikely that the ideal CIS will be available on the market. Trying to imagine the ideal system in concrete terms and being both realistic and adventurous will help when considering choices and trade-offs.

Making choices

Viewing systems in action in other units provides an opportunity to move beyond imagining what a CIS might do. It allows understanding of how it performs in key tasks, such as providing data during ward rounds, producing forms, or extracting data. It can reveal the work that may be needed to achieve the envisioned capabilities.

Taking this kind of hands-on approach to the decision-making process will help shape the vision of the ideal CIS. It is more likely that claims made regarding the CIS will be accurate and transparent.

Making trade-offs

Along with choices will come trade-offs.

Some trade-offs may be particular to the combination of criteria, such as the need for a customizable user interface to match the workflow and the desire to have an off-the-shelf system.

Commercial systems will rarely fulfil each criterion to the same degree so choice depends on relative importance of criteria.

It is possible to do a formal decision analysis by determining criteria and their weights, giving each system a score per criterion, and summing up the weighted scores across all criteria. Some criteria may be difficult to get firm evidence on or may not be easily quantifiable. It may be just as useful to identify criteria and relative importance without doing a formal calculation. This can be helpful in clarifying expectations and trade-offs involved for all of stakeholders.

Other trade-offs are inherent to group working and are more difficult. If the system creates less work for one person, it may well create more for others. For example, an information system can make data collection for management decisions easy, but create more disruptions in the clinical workflow at the bedside.

It is important to identify all the stakeholders and engage representatives from each group in the CIS selection process. Setting up working groups to examine specific topics relevant to their work can encourage this engagement. Trade-offs cannot be avoided, but they can be done thoughtfully.

Software choice

Every critical care unit operates differently, which means that the CIS software needs to be adapted to the unit or that the unit needs to adapt to the CIS software.

In reality, it is likely that both will happen as these are two extremes on a continuum.

The most significant decision for choosing CIS software is determining the amount and type of customization of the software to adapt it to your unit and its way of working.

Customizing a CIS

It can be easy to believe that local circumstances are so individual as to be supportable only by a bespoke CIS specifically designed to meet them.

However, the problems experienced in developing systems from scratch, and the expense of maintaining and upgrading them, means that a bespoke CIS for an individual unit is now very rarely a viable financial solution.

The other end of the spectrum is the commercial 'off-the-shelf' CIS. Seeking to maximize their potential market, vendors usually want to make their systems as universal as possible requiring that a unit adapts its processes to the CIS. As few units are willing to do this, there is often opportunity for customization.

Consequently, the significant decision in purchasing a CIS is not whether to get a bespoke system or an off-the-shelf one, but rather the amount of customization required for an off-the-shelf CIS and who does it.

Most commercially available CIS software is customizable, some extensively. Deciding on the amount of customization will depend on needs of the unit and ability of staff to tolerate mismatches between software and work practices. Although there may be significant pressures towards extensive customization of a CIS, the greater the degree of customization the greater the cost.

Customization requires devoting resources to carry out the customization as well as to maintain the changes, potentially needing to reapply the customizations every time the system is upgraded. As there will always be some degree of mismatch between the design of the system and the specific requirements of an individual unit, the amount of customization will be a balance between needs and cost.

Most systems are customized by consulting software engineers, who will need to be given requirements at the start of the project.

Some systems now allow users (or a small subset of them, designated super-users) to do customization. In the latter case, the super-user is supplied with a large number of building blocks and given the capability to put them together in a way that suits the unit. The analogy is to building with LEGO® blocks.

This possibility of the user doing the customization may be restricted to the user interface or may extend to doing sophisticated jobs such as building a database or reports.

Selecting professionals or end-users to customize offers different possibilities for the customization of the system and its later development.

There are advantages and disadvantages to both approaches. If the customization is done by consulting software engineers then the system does not require substantial clinical time to carry out the customization. On the other hand, the requirements for the customization need to be set before the system is used. Although this may seem relatively straightforward, it is extremely difficult to predict how people will use the system before they have tried it.

When customization is done by users, it can be done as and when necessary. For example, one unit decided that they needed a new button to reach a nursing form more quickly and the super-user did this in a matter of minutes. The same change could have taken days or weeks and incurred a fee if it had been done by consultant software engineers.

This almost instant customization is a bonus when trying to win the 'hearts and minds' of the team, as perceived mistakes can be rectified quickly and suggestions implemented with little delay. In the first few weeks post-implementation, this instant response is essential to maintain staff confidence in the system – there is nothing worse than introducing a new system that is then not fit-for-purpose in some respects, but cannot be readily altered.

Box 4.1

One unit discovered that a small discrepancy in how some fluid prescriptions were set led to fluid balances being incorrect – this caused enormous angst amongst both medical and nursing staff but, once identified, it was quickly rectified by a user trained in customization, and confidence in the CIS was greatly improved.

Box 4.2

Visiting surgeons were opposed to the introduction of a CIS in a specific unit and criticized the inability to have the information they needed in one location as it meant having to scroll through screens of information. It took only 30 minutes for an end-user to work with a surgeon to design a page that had all the data they required, immediately increasing acceptance of the CIS by other groups.

A further advantage of user-customization is that it allows the clinical staff to experiment with and introduce process improvements or new ways of working.

Process improvements might facilitate clinical work at the bedside by integrating the data collection forms with the way that nurses work. Small changes of the system can provide a mechanism for introducing and monitoring the use of new guidelines. The ability to change parts of the system quickly supports the development of clinical practice over time as the information system becomes embedded in the clinical environment. Such flexibility would be too costly if done by software engineers.

The disadvantage of user-customization is that it takes significant clinical time of a few select people and may involve learning a specialized tool or programming language. The system is highly dependent on the knowledge of the local customizers, which can cause problems if they leave and do not document their work.

The authors of this book advocate the use of user-customizable systems if there is the clinical time available to maintain them.

Regardless of whether customization is done within the unit or by software engineers, it is important to probe the scope of possible customization work if significant customization is envisaged. Every system will have aspects that are fundamental to its structure and cannot be changed. Identifying these in

Table 4.2 Common criteria

Cost
System reliability and performance
Ease of use
Functionality
Security
Reputation of vendor

advance provides the opportunity to check that they are compatible with unit practices.

It is important to budget appropriately for customization work. This includes planning for customization before implementation as well as throughout the life of the system, ensuring that adequate clinical time is available to determine the requirements.

Long-term buy-in by management at the organizational level is necessary to ensure that the support for release of staff time continues. Experience shows that the initial enthusiasm to this commitment can wane over time when the system becomes embedded in an organization – this means that change takes longer to occur, leading to a less responsive system. It can lead to a reliance on the goodwill of the customizers to continue developments, sometimes on top of existing workload and in their own time.

Common criteria

Alongside the decision about the amount of customization and who does it, there are common criteria that are usually considered when selecting an information system such as a CIS. These are listed in Table 4.2.

Cost is likely to be a significant factor in choice. The total cost, not just the cost of the software, needs to be calculated and considered.

The system's reliability and performance are important and can be evaluated for back-up mechanisms and previous history.

Ease of use can be determined by having a range of proposed system users trying the system.

Functionality and security needs will need to align with unit work practices and local standards.

The reputation for the vendor should be considered. Are the vendors established and likely to be around in ten years' time to continue to upgrade your system? Do they have a reputation for being helpful and supportive? Choosing a vendor is much like interviewing for a new colleague and needs to consider the long term.

Hardware

There is a large (and growing) variety of IT equipment that can be used to deliver a CIS in critical care settings.

Devices

A choice needs to be made about the devices on which to run the CIS. In critical care settings where patients are typically immobile and receive individual care, a standard set-up is to have a computer at every bedside, supplemented by computers elsewhere on the unit, or even off it, to access the

CIS. Depending on the setting, more mobility than this may be desirable.

Fixed devices, such as a desktop computer, have numerous advantages. They tend to be cheaper, are less likely to be damaged, and often provide larger screens.

Finding somewhere to locate a fixed device may be a problem if suitable work surfaces are scarce. As space around the bedside may be at a premium, it may be necessary to be able to move the device out of the way at times. The installation of computers on movable carts, or on a wall-mounted arm, may be a compromise solution in such situations.

Mobile devices can be carried around by staff and come in a variety of forms.

Laptop computers can often provide similar, or even equivalent, functionality to desktop computers, but to make them reasonably mobile they usually have smaller screens. This is most likely to be an issue if more than one person needs to view the screen. Laptops require a work surface at a convenient height for the user. This can be achieved by fitting them to a trolley (a so-called computer on wheels, or COW, as shown in Figure 4.1).

Another mobile option is a tablet PC with touch screen and pen-like stylus for data entry (Figure 4.2). These may be most suitable for use when standing and large amounts of free text entry are not required. This model can be useful, for example, on ward rounds, allowing one member of the team to document daily plans, amend prescriptions and order tests at the time of the round, without disrupting the viewing of information on a central monitor. Speed should be checked to ensure it is fast enough for the proposed task.

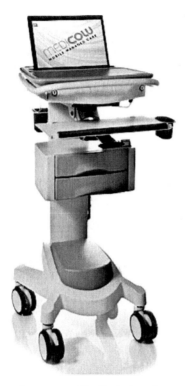

Figure 4.1 Computer on a specifically designed ergonomic cart. (Adapted with permission from Medicow.co.uk)

Portable devices face a number of practical considerations. They need to be robust to survive drops or falls and have adequate battery life to last through all tasks before recharging. Carrying convenience, i.e. of suitable size to fit in a pocket, should be considered. It is essential to have a plan that motivates staff to remember to recharge devices and not walk

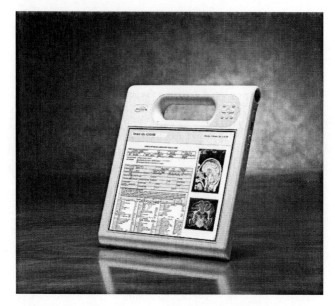

Figure 4.2 Portable computer. (Adapted with permission from Medicow.co.uk)

off with them in their pockets, inadvertently or otherwise. If devices do not fit in a pocket, a strategy for carrying them while performing clinical activities will need to be created.

Box 4.3

Allied health professionals were eager to have a portable device so that they could review data at the bedside during ward rounds. This proved possible only for the first 10 patients of the unit as the weight of the device strained the users' shoulders.

Table 4.3 Advantages and disadvantages of various devices

Device	Screen size	Portability	Functionality	Other issues
Desktop computer	Large	No	Full	Space at bedside
Laptop	Medium	Yes	Full	Use when standing, weight
Tablet PC	Medium	Yes	Full	Cost, slower data entry via touch screen
Netbook	Small	Yes	Full	Small keyboard and screen, use when standing
PDA/Smartphone	Small	Yes	Limited	Data entry, screen size

When making trade-offs between devices, screen size is particularly important to consider. Larger screens will be needed to view detailed text and figures. This is particularly true if more than one person needs to view them at the same time, such as when discussing a result. The viewing angle should be considered. Even large screens may have a limit to the number of people who can view the screen simultaneously, which could affect ward round participation. Lighting conditions affect what can be seen on the screen. It is difficult to read screens in bright light, such as near a window. Careful consideration should therefore be given to the type and positioning of screens to suit the working conditions and practices in the unit.

Table 4.3 summarizes the advantages and disadvantages of various types of fixed and mobile devices.

Data entry devices

When an appropriate computer has been chosen, consideration needs to be given to choosing supporting data entry devices, such as keyboards and mice.

Data entry devices can be a source of infection. Washable or disposable keyboards and mice are one means of infection control, but they are more expensive and are often considered less responsive because the keys are covered by a washable membrane.

Washable keyboards and mice may not be ideal if strong encouragement to use the system is needed, as they may discourage CIS use.

Cables connecting mice and keyboards to the computer may be another potential source of contamination. This can be avoided with the use of wireless devices, although the reliability, connectivity and battery life of such devices may create other difficulties.

Further issues that may arise are the robustness of data entry devices, which may get spilled on or knocked around; the visibility of keyboards when used at night (see Figure 4.3: a black keyboard is a problem in critical care when lights are dimmed at night but data entered at all times); and the availability of suitable surfaces on which to operate a mouse.

There are no easy solutions. It is recommended that devices are tested for a time to ascertain their robustness and appropriateness in your environment.

It may be necessary to get equipment of clinical grade to meet regulations.

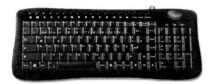

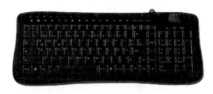

Figure 4.3 A black and white keyboard may look smart in daylight but the keys will be invisible to your night staff.

Networks, power and printers

A less immediately visible aspect of hardware choice is the types of network and power supplies for CIS devices.

The choice regarding networks is largely whether to go for a wired or wireless system. The cost, reliability and speed of wireless networks have been steadily improving, and concerns about interference with medical equipment have been largely resolved.

Careful planning of the location of wireless access points is necessary to ensure complete coverage of an area. Where the CIS is accessed through fixed devices, then wired networks may be the better option. Planning is required so that the computer is most appropriately placed for the user and not put wherever the network connection is found.

Original solutions such as umbilical cords can be designed. Figure 4.4 shows such a solution in place.

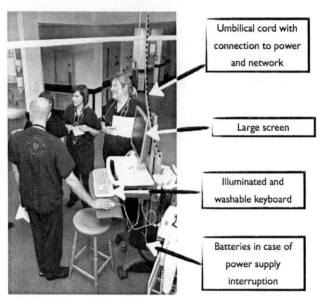

Figure 4.4

Choices have to be made even with power supplies, the options being mains power or batteries. A consideration with the use of mains power may be the number of available plug sockets in settings where there is already a large amount of equipment, but this generally remains the cheaper and more reliable option unless mobile devices are widely used for CIS access. Battery-powered devices will be constrained by the duration of battery life and by whether users remember to recharge them.

If on the mains, the hardware should be connected to the back-up electrical supply to ensure continuity of care. This should include all elements of the system, not just the computers used at the bedside.

Printers are usually required. CIS is often presented as leading to paperless documentation, but it is unlikely that paper and printers can be eliminated. Printers may still be necessary for devices that cannot be integrated with the CIS: to print records for discharge of patients to settings that do not have access to the CIS; and to create essential documentation in the case of partial system failure.

If the CIS is not well matched to their specific clinical workflows, staff may want to be able to print out data to make their own documentation, such as patient or 'to do' lists.

Removing all access to printers may lead to the proliferation of informal documentation with increased risk of transcription errors.

There is a good case for limiting printing from a CIS as the evidence suggests that paper usage often increases with the introduction of computers. Emails or multiple drafts of documents are printed, for example. Restrictions on who can print and what can be printed from the CIS may be necessary.

The layout of output from a CIS may lead to inefficient use of paper and this should be addressed.

Server

A number of the benefits of a CIS come from the creation of a central data repository. Paper forms can only be in one place at one time, whereas data in a CIS can be viewed from different locations simultaneously. A member of staff no longer has to be at the bedside to view a patient's record.

Further, data previously on separate paper forms can be collated and compared over time in a CIS and previous records are easily retrievable and searchable. In order for this to be possible, records need to be held on a central server, a powerful computer that feeds the devices and computers that staff access.

There are various ways in which a server can be configured.

One particularly relevant choice for healthcare professionals is between what are called 'thick' and 'thin' clients.

A thick client has the user interface, applications and the data most likely to be used all stored on the computer from which the CIS is accessed and uses the server to back-up data and store data less frequently accessed, such as old charts.

Thin clients have only the interface on the local computer; all applications and data are stored on the server.

Each type of client has advantages and disadvantages.

The advantage of a thick client is the resilience it provides if there are problems with the server or network. It may speed up access to applications and data if the network is slow or congested.

Thin clients facilitate system administration and upgrades, enable greater security and make more efficient use of computer resources. Thin client devices are typically cheaper than thick client ones.

In practice, server clients may lie somewhere in between these two extremes and the extent to which the advantages of either model are realized may depend on local circumstances, for example hardware purchasing or security policies.

Login

The need to login is an essential element of the way that CIS works.

It ensures the confidentiality of patient records, and allows only authorised personnel to view or enter particular data or orders. It couples actions in the CIS with an individual who is then responsible.

The login mechanism can be a source of great frustration to staff. Compared with the use of paper records, logins introduce an additional step in accessing and using the CIS that users may come across many times during a working day.

There are various ways of logging in to a CIS. The most common is the use of usernames and passwords. Effort should be made to ensure that usernames are short so that people are not discouraged from logging in many times.

The system should easily give new staff usernames and allow them to set their passwords. All staff need to have access to password reminders (especially if they work irregular hours with long interruptions).

Logging out should require a single key-stroke, and users should be consistently reminded about its importance, as they could be liable for any actions carried out under their own login.

The system must log people out after a period of inactivity.

The system should encourage staff to change their passwords regularly for security purposes but systems that block access are not desirable as they are likely to affect the ability to deliver care.

Other means of identifying users are swipe cards, keys or proximity devices.

Swipe cards allow users to login quickly to the CIS, to view patient data for example, without using the keyboard. This may be an effective system if staff already have swipe cards, as it eliminates the problem of assigning usernames and ensuring passwords are remembered and secure.

Keys are similar but stay in a device next to the computer while the user is signed in. They have the advantage of being fast and of encouraging the user to logout (by taking their key) when they are finished, increasing security.

Proximity devices are made active when a person comes close to the computer, making them a hands-free way to login. These are particularly convenient for users and ensure automatic logout, but may be problematic if there are several people using the computer, or the user is going back and forth between the bed and computer and constantly being logged out.

Swipe cards, keys and proximity devices often make CIS usage easier, but increase costs. They do not necessarily increase security as the system recognizes the card, key or device and not the user.

Devices can be shared as easily as a username and password. To try to prevent such security threats, sharing access can be made a disciplinary offence. However, on its own this is unlikely to be effective. For example, senior staff who are unwilling to use a keyboard or consider that using the CIS takes too long to enable them to get their work done may request junior staff to use the CIS for them.

Provision may be considered to allow users to indicate that they are using a CIS on the instruction of another staff member.

A similar issue may arise with staff who are only visiting and for whom the overhead of creating and maintaining a user account may be high (including training on how to use the system). The provision of 'guest' or 'supervised' accounts with limited capabilities may be considered.

Device interconnectivity

Critical care units are technology-intensive areas. Consequently a CIS used in critical care must be able to communicate both to and from all other relevant systems and devices.

Other devices include other clinical information systems or electronic patient records used by related units (e.g. wards, general practices) as well as machines such as ventilators and monitors.

Additionally, the unit may be responsible for giving data to management or government bodies. In the UK, for example, every critical care unit must provide the Critical Care Minimum Data Set (CCMDS) to the government.

It is key to think about device interconnectivity before buying a CIS.

It is important to consider how data are output from the CIS. While a pdf might look nice and be useful for printing a report, it will make it difficult to collate the data in different ways for government bodies or other purposes such as research. Data that are in a raw form from a database, on the other hand, may require high levels of programming expertise to extract and to manipulate them (and don't look nice.).

Data may need to meet certain clinical coding standards, such as the international healthcare informatics interoperability standards HL7, and the CIS should support this.

Certain data requirements may be the same across a large number of units, owing to government regulation, for example, and units should coordinate to ensure that vendors support them.

Communication between devices, particularly software such as CIS or electronic patient records, is necessary to achieve integrated working of the CIS.

Conversely, it is equally important that the data are secure and not so easily movable that they can be taken out of the unit.

USB ports and emails are common ways that information can be copied from the system. USB ports might need to be disabled on, and personal emails made inaccessible from, devices on which the CIS is accessed.

Collaboration with the IT department is required to ensure that patient data are secured without causing extreme inconvenience to legitimate needs of staff, such as having a printout of their patients' relevant data.

Work is needed around information governance training for all staff to ensure that confidential information is treated in accordance with local policy.

Connecting to other hardware devices in the unit, such as ventilators, is a challenging device interconnectivity problem. It is necessary to check whether the device can connect, that the relevant driver – the piece of software that allows two particular devices to communicate – is available or will be written, and that appropriate outlet ports are installed.

Each device will probably need a different driver and perhaps a different plug. This can be a costly process so it is best to explore the needs early on. It means that it can be expensive to change or upgrade other technology in the unit.

Rigorous checks are required early on to ensure that the devices will actually communicate and not just look as though they will communicate.

Box 4.4

A new syringe has been developed for use in critical care. It has a port for connecting to a CIS. When probed whether it worked and whether the drivers, or software, were in place, it was discovered that these ports were not connected to anything inside the pump. Although the device looked as though it would communicate, on further inspection it was found that it would not.

Claims by the vendors of the ability of devices to communicate are not always realized in practice – always ask to see the systems working before committing to purchase.

Table 4.4 is a scorecard adapted from one designed by Kim French (MHSA, CAPPM) and Edward Diamond. Other units

Table 4.4 Vendor selection scorecard

Adapted by permission from Kim D. French, MHSA, CAPPM

Score:			
0 = Not applicable/observed			
1 = Does not meet expectation			
2 = Meets expectation			
3 = Exceeds expectation			
Attribute	Vendor A	Vendor B	Vendor C

Support

Response time to calls

Hours of support operations (weekend/night?)

Onsite or web-based support and training

Quarterly product updates

Annual product updates

Hourly support charges

Support of existing systems/products

Annual maintenance pricing

Connectivity outsourced or insourced

Subtotal

Hardware

Hardware compatibility

Internet/Intranet

Technology base

Handheld/mobile/remote options

Scanners

Imaging into the database

Imaging into attachments

Automatic back-up

Server redundancy (downtime prevention)

Application Service Provider (ASP) or
   on-demand software model available

Open architecture

Table 4.4 (*cont.*)

Attribute	Vendor A	Vendor B	Vendor C

Subtotal

Software

Windows

Relational database

Product interface options

Date, time, user stamp options

Ease of system navigation (windows and clicks)

Subtotal

Scheduling

Manages multiple resources

Manages multiple sites

Click and drag appointments

Summary screen of appointments in scheduler

Automated wait listing

Scheduling hot button (on the fly)

Easy overrides and template changes

Compatible with phone tree etc

Subtotal

Billing functions

Electronic claims

Electronic remits

Clearinghouse interfaces

Statement generation

Charge entry and numbers of clicks

Batch posting by exception

Encounter tracking to scheduler

Managed care / referral module

Collections module

Annual update

Interface

Claims scrub to electronic record

(*cont.*)

Table 4.4 (*cont.*)

Attribute	Vendor A	Vendor B	Vendor C
Subtotal			
Workflow			
Patient tracking during visits			
Patient tracking during phone triage			
Electronic messaging between physicians/staff			
Tracks interval services – schedules from there			
Templates on demand			
Lab interface			
Patient editor built in and automatically recorded			
Treatment management with formularies			
Treatment management with allergies/reactions/side effects			
Prescription process			
Graphic report options			
Physician quality reporting initiative			
Support national care guidelines			
Reduces/automates staff time			
Voice recognition			
Subtotal			
Reporting			
Dashboard management reports			
Realtime utilization reporting			
User defined and templated			
Extraction of clinical data			
Create letters and documents			
Benchmark outcomes against guidelines			
Fax/email directly			
Subtotal			
Total vendor score			

might find it a useful starting point for considering different software.

Key points

- Choosing a CIS involves a multitude of decisions.
- Building a picture of the ideal system will help to navigate through the decisions about software, hardware and device interconnectivity.
- Decisions will require the involvement of a range of different staff and it is helpful to set up working groups to examine particular topics, such as device connectivity, input devices or data output standards.
- Hardware requires a lot of input from those who will be using it to ensure that the ergonomics are suitable.

TO LEARN MORE

E. Diamond, K. French, C. Gronkiewicz and M. Borkgren, 2010. Electronic medical records, *Chest* 138(3): 716–23. doi:10.1378/chest.09–1328.

Chapter 5

Planning for success

Introduction

The key to successful implementation is a coherent strategy.

The first section of this chapter, 'Planning for implementation', discusses the details that should be considered before commencing the implementation process.

With the increased activity around implementation, monitoring its effects is often overlooked.

The second section, 'Monitoring implementation', details the steps that should be taken to monitor the implementation process.

When planning for success it is important to plan for problems, ensuring that contingency plans are in place that can be readily implemented if any aspect of the CIS or supporting hardware stops functioning.

The final section of this chapter, 'Planning for problems', details the most common problems likely to be encountered and describes possible contingencies.

Planning for implementation

Discussion of the go-live date, the first day CIS will be used in a unit, is likely to generate fear as well as excitement. There are many small details to plan and a host of potential problems. Having a well-thought-through plan can take some of the anxiety out of the anticipation of the go-live date.

As with any project management, identify all activities that need to take place before and during implementation and their expected duration.

Identify dependencies between activities and the critical pathway (the sequence of activities that will be slowest and will therefore determine the length of a project). It may be helpful to draw a timeline of these activities and highlight dependencies in red. Alternatively, use standard project management software, such as Microsoft Visio, to create a Gantt chart that illustrates the relationships between activities.

Once the dependencies are clear, any risks arising from delays can be determined. For example, if training has been planned once the customization is finished and there is a significant delay in the customization at the last minute, the training budget could be lost unless training is switched to a generic version of the system.

Recording the sequence of events and their duration will help determine the time that will be needed to carry out pre- and post-implementation activities. A rule of thumb in software engineering is that the amount of time that something is expected to take should be doubled to get the actual time required. A cautious project leader might triple the expected time.

Pilot environment

Regardless of the implementation approach, having a pilot environment is good practice. It allows the waters to be tested before rolling out the system. Pilots can identify any mismatches between the CIS and current clinical practices.

A pilot environment can locate any obvious software bugs and integration issues. For example, it could be discovered that the software interface between the ventilator and the CIS causes the CIS to stop working. Such problems can occur because the two pieces of software have probably been made by different vendors and the link between the two may have been only simulated, rather than tested in practice.

The scale of a pilot depends on the scale of the full implementation. If the implementation is in one unit, the pilot may be carried out with just a few beds. If the implementation is hospital-wide, a pilot may consist of implementing the system in full in one unit.

Pilots are useful in identifying problems, and are easier to stop if things go wrong. They have a strong demonstration effect that helps staff really understand what their environment will be like once they are using the CIS.

It must be kept in mind that pilots often mean that temporary interfaces are needed to areas not involved in the pilot and that system benefits may not reveal themselves in their entirety.

Implementation strategy

Once a pilot is completed, the implementation strategy will need to be decided. The two extremes are doing everything in one go, a so-called 'big bang' strategy, or to phase the system in over time. In reality, most units will have a strategy that sits between these.

The 'big bang' approach involves implementing the CIS with all beds (or units) at the same time. This has numerous advantages, including no need for temporary interfaces between systems or to maintain and update legacy systems. It allows staff to have a first impression of the system as it will be. They will not need to deal with functionality links not working, for example. This approach suggests to staff that there is no going back to the old system, reducing the risk of revolt. Moreover, as the implementation time is shorter, the cost is likely to be less.

This approach has disadvantages as well. It requires a large peak of resources which may be difficult to manage and will probably lead to fewer resources across all (sub-)units. The demonstration effect is not as dramatic and the development time might be longer.

At the other extreme is a phased implementation, which means the implementation is done in stages. These stages could relate to number of beds or units, or to functionality. For example, a unit may implement the documentation part of a CIS first and implement drug prescribing when staff have adjusted to the system. This approach requires fewer peak resources and gives staff time to learn the systems, and may improve the engagement of staff who were previously sceptical. In addition, there is the back-up of the legacy system if the CIS falls flat.

The disadvantages are that there will be heavy use of temporary interfaces to make the whole system fit together. Staff may find this annoying or, worse, frustrating, as the interaction will not have been designed and the temporary interfaces are likely to have software bugs because they will not have been thoroughly tested.

The cost of a phased approach will be higher than the 'big bang' approach, because of the need to maintain legacy systems, create temporary interfaces and have support staff on hand for a longer period.

With a phased approach, there is the risk that the full implementation will never happen. This could be seen in a positive light as it could suggest that people stopped an inappropriate system before it was too late. It is more likely that a failure to fully implement the system reflects a lack of resources or confidence to continue. As a result staff will never see the full benefits of the system. This is the worst of all: staff do not like the system, it does not function well, and it is costly.

Units that have the capacity and strong clinical leadership but may be at risk of staff rejecting the new system are probably best to follow a 'big bang' approach.

Those concerned about high staff stress or capacity may choose a phased approach.

In reality, most units will have an approach somewhere between these two extremes.

One compromise is to implement the CIS at beds with new patients. In that way, it is naturally phased in over a period of weeks, not months. There are no arbitrary deadlines to argue about.

Box 5.1

One unit decided to go for the 'big bang' approach. Changing all existing patients to the CIS proved difficult and the easiest solution was to go for an approach by which any new patient admitted to the unit was on the CIS, while any patient who had been present before remained on paper. Within a few weeks, all patients' records were solely electronic.

Implementation contingency plans

A complete implementation plan will include realistic contingencies in case there are problems and/or delays.

In practice contingency plans are sometimes exhausted. One approach is to not tell anyone, press on, and hope to meet the original deadline. This is unlikely to lead to success. Not only will it increase the stress on the development team, there is also the risk that corners are cut. This is likely to generate anger when the system goes live and does not function as expected.

It is possible to reduce the scope and do only a partial implementation. This carries the risk that significant functionality and performance will be lost and possibly never recovered.

A more productive response is to postpone the go-live date. The earlier this can be done the less damage in terms of committed costs, such as booked extra staff, and the less likely it is that pessimistic rumours will spread.

If a postponement is necessary, a realistic new date should be set (twice as far away as when the software is expected to be completed). Postponing twice will do even more damage, and projects postponed three times are unlikely to survive.

Progress of the system should be reported to the staff and reasons for any delays explained. If the need to get the system right to support staff work practices and patient safety is emphasized, most staff will be understanding.

Planning for after go-live

When planning implementation, the period after go-live requires as much consideration as before it. For example, more support staff are likely to be needed than was expected. Trainers should be on the unit 24 hours a day for at least the first week.

It is helpful to have supernumerary staff to ease workloads.

Before deciding to reduce support, review levels of stress and staff morale.

Staff who are having particular difficulties should be identified and assigned someone with more confidence to establish the reasons for their problems and provide appropriate support.

Monitoring implementation

It can be easy to get wrapped up in the day-to-day demands of implementation and lose sight of the overall picture.

It is important to monitor the implementation to ensure that all problems, not just software ones, are addressed. For example, a CIS can affect ward round communication. It is important to recognize that this is happening and look for possible solutions. If there is a need to show the benefits of the CIS, appropriate data will need to be collected.

In this section we discuss several ways that implementation can be monitored. This section is meant to be a reminder to ensure a monitoring process is in place before the project gets caught up in the pressures of implementation.

Baseline data

In order to identify and demonstrate effects of CIS implementation, it will be necessary to record and benchmark pre-CIS practices as a reference point. This will allow evidence to be gathered to assess claims of improvement from CIS proponents or of deterioration from CIS opponents. Such evidence might include time spent on patient care or CIS use, or documentation of processes and problems, including use of guidelines, medication errors, calculation and transcription errors. Inefficiencies that the CIS is expected to remove should also be captured.

These suggested areas from which to capture evidence are likely to be familiar to any healthcare professional who reads research papers. It is important to consider issues raised by staff.

Anonymous questionnaires can be used to monitor staff morale and attitudes toward CIS, while interviews may be the best forum for staff to present concerns and overarching problems with CIS. Not only will this provide the implementation team with valuable insight to improve implementation efforts and communication strategies; staff might appreciate the opportunity to express themselves, particularly if they perceive that suggestions will be acted upon.

It is important to gather the benchmark data well before implementation to avoid findings being influenced by the implementation activities. It is recommended that the data be gathered at least one month prior to training.

Studies that look at staff attitudes and concerns should be started closer to the implementation date so that views are informed by a realistic understanding of the system. As a reality check, it is helpful to benchmark against practices in other hospitals or other units in the same hospital to identify local (in)efficiencies.

Third party monitoring

In the tumult of implementation planning, it can be difficult to find the time to gather data. It may be helpful to have an external third party monitor implementation, perhaps from a local university.

University researchers may be particularly appropriate to investigate staff views and concerns which staff may not want to express to colleagues. They can bring new perspectives and challenge taken-for-granted assumptions. University researchers may see the implementation as a whole from an outsider's perspective and comment on phenomena that can be difficult to see from the inside.

Box 5.2

One hospital brought in a multidisciplinary team of researchers from the fields of information systems, psychology, anthropology and computer science to assess its implementation strategy and be an outside eye. The team looked at staff morale, staff concerns with implementation, the impact of CIS on communication patterns in the ward round, and user-customization. The research team fed back regularly to the implementation steering group as well as publishing several research papers.

Issue log

Establishing benchmark data and asking a third party to monitor the implementation will not usually capture CIS-specific issues, such as 'there needs to be a button to the drug chart on the ward round screen'. An issue log is a good way to capture these. It can be part of the CIS if it is customizable, or it can be in a notebook or large whiteboard that everyone has easy access to. Until staff become comfortable with the CIS, the latter option may be better received as it will be a more familiar mode of communication.

Such a log provides an outlet for concerns and is a way to acknowledge some of the difficulties that staff might be facing when using the system. It is important to review and respond rapidly to issues that arise as well as to highlight positive changes made.

Box 5.3

One unit developed an online form that people could fill out that was accompanied by a list of noted problems and responses. This gave people a sense of satisfaction that their problems were dealt with and reduced the number of duplicate problems being entered.

Planning for problems

As the CIS will be the main repository of all data regarding patient care when it is fully operational, it is essential to have contingency plans in place in the event of a system failure or other disaster.

Each will be considered in turn with their specific solutions before discussing the creation of robust contingency plans.

Power

Without power the CIS server and devices cannot function and consequently no access to the CIS will be possible.

Power could be lost hospital-wide, unit-wide, or just to a particular device, so it is important to consider what back-up power supplies can be deployed in each case and how quickly.

If the hospital has a generator, ensure it can support the power needs of the CIS in addition to the rest of the hospital. It may be necessary to buy a generator specifically for the unit, or a CIS that can run in a reduced mode during power outages.

Every unit should have a paper back-up system in case of multiple failures. Some CIS systems support such back-up, with the ability to print recent crucial information (e.g. medications) to facilitate care on paper.

The server is a device that needs particular thought as it is crucial to the CIS working properly. If it runs on a different power supply from the CIS, it will require its own alternative power supply as a back-up. It is necessary to ensure that the server (which will run unattended for most of the time) is not accidentally switched off as the significance of this may not be immediately evident.

> **Box 5.4**
>
> Despite having servers and computers with back-up power supply, one hospital experienced a major CIS failure when a cleaner unplugged the CIS server to get a free power socket for a vacuum cleaner.

A duplicate copy of the information stored on the server should be kept on the same power supply as the unit if this is not interruptible. This is particularly important if a 'thin client' is being used and all applications and data are stored remotely. If the server is duplicated it is necessary to have a transition plan from one copy to the other so that it can be done smoothly in an emergency.

Network failures

Network failures can cause significant disruption and can be difficult to fix.

'Thin clients' and wireless systems are more susceptible to network problems and this trade-off should be considered when choosing them.

Wireless systems should have back-up routers that can be changed quickly with the option to plug into a network if necessary.

The weakest point of a network is often at an unexpected location.

Hardware failures

Hardware failures will occur, but are easy to fix if suitable preparations are in place. Devices break for a multitude of reasons. They could be faulty, or be dropped or damaged in other ways.

Cleaning with inappropriate products is often a problem as screens and keyboards will be irreversibly damaged by some chemicals.

Spare devices should be readily available so users can replace those damaged without calling the IT department or a senior CIS manager.

If a particular device is consistently being broken, the quality of the equipment and the specific area of use should be reviewed.

A lack of space on the working surface for the keyboard will cause it to be continually dropped. In that case, the working surface should be adapted rather than the keyboard.

Critical care is a busy environment and devices will get broken more quickly than one might expect in a home or regular office. This will need to be planned for in the budget. In one unit, keyboards and mice are damaged every couple of weeks and screens need replacing at least once a year.

The most problematic hardware failure is the server as it stores all the data that the unit has accumulated. It is important to back-up the server regularly, just as it is with a personal computer. Once a week is a standard interval to back-up a server, but this will depend on the type of CIS in use and the value of the data.

Software failure

Total software failures are unlikely for a CIS that is established on the market.

CIS are complicated systems that are frequently being updated and some 'bugs' or unexpected behaviour of the system are expected.

Software engineers recognize that no amount of testing will catch all bugs, so vendors across industries aim to catch only the majority of bugs before release and expect to fix other bugs as they arise.

Safety-critical systems, such as a CIS on which people's lives depend, will be developed in such a way that the risk of safety-critical failures is minimized.

It is important to report software bugs to the software vendor. For the report to be helpful, it will need to record the conditions of failure. These include whether the problem is recurrent or transient, whether there are any known reproducible triggers (e.g. using the print function from a specific page) and what the outcome is (e.g. the computer freezes). Once these have been noted, the vendor should be informed through the bug reporting system that most CIS vendors have.

Sometimes vendors will identify a bug as a 'known problem' (i.e. one that they do not consider to be a priority for resolution). Known problems are likely to relate to fundamental characteristics of the software design that cannot be easily changed. If this is the case, it is important to emphasize the clinical impact of a bug to guide the vendors in allocating resources to fix issues.

Robust contingency plans

Contingency plans for when the CIS goes down consist of two elements: the activities that can be done routinely to decrease the degree of the failure and the plan that is in place when disaster strikes.

Back-up of all system data should be done routinely from the server. The frequency depends on the acceptable level of data loss and this should be defined before implementation. If data are lost for a month, week or day, what problems would this create? Who would face these problems?

If archived clinical data are lost, for example, the only person affected is likely to be a future researcher. If data used for billing are lost, a week's loss might be of concern to the accounts department, depending on the frequency with which they collect their data.

Fortunately, the datasets, even after several years of use, are normally gigabytes rather than terabytes, so are not difficult to back-up frequently.

To decide upon the optimal amount of data to back-up, consider all stakeholders that would be affected if the data were lost. Note that different data may need to be backed-up at different rates. Current patient data may need to be backed-up hourly, and archived data once a week.

It is common to have multiple back-ups, to provide some redundancy in case one back-up becomes corrupt.

Location of the back-up is important. A unit should have at least one local copy in case the network or an off-site server goes down but the unit does not.

Back-up procedures must be discussed with the vendor, as they are likely to have some in place and may even hold a copy of customers' servers.

Once a regular back-up plan is in place, it is important to monitor it. Check that the back-up is taking place and that the system restores properly. Likely back-up problems to guard against are the data becoming corrupted and therefore unusable; the most recent data being restored but not parts of the archive; and all functionality not operating correctly.

In addition to back-ups it is necessary to have a plan of action that can be put in place when a failure occurs. This plan should have varying levels of escalation depending on the expected duration of the outage, its location and its extent. If the outage occurs and the expectation from those who have located it is that it will only be a few minutes, then nothing needs to be done. If it is a few hours, an alternative strategy will be needed.

Staff should be aware of what the contingency plans are and how to activate them. These should be shown at induction for new starters.

In a worst case scenario, many critical care units with a CIS have emergency packs of paper forms that can be used in conjunction with an emergency set of data that can be printed locally from the CIS even when not functioning. This may be easy to implement just after the transition from paper, but will get progressively more difficult as staff are employed on the unit who have not used the paper documentation. One unit noted that people who had used paper for 20 years found it difficult to switch back. Their way of thinking about data had changed to fit the CIS and was no longer in line with the paper. If paper is part of the contingency plan, ensure that staff are regularly trained in its use. The form of the paper documentation may have to be adapted as complex charts will not be understood by staff who are used to electronic documentation.

Key points

- The best way to plan for success is to have a well-thought-out implementation strategy and monitoring program.
- Have robust contingency plans in place.
- Use a team approach in managing the implementation and ensure that adequate clinical time has been allocated to the tasks.

TO LEARN MORE

N. C. Nelson, 2007. Downtime procedures for a clinical information system: a critical issue, *Journal of Critical Care* 22(1): 45–50. doi:10.1016/j.jcrc.2007.01.004.

Chapter 6

Training

Introduction

Training is an essential part of implementing a CIS and needs considerable attention to ensure success. It achieves a level of familiarity with the system that engages staff in the possibilities the system offers, reduces the learning curve during clinical time and identifies potential problems or difficulties at a time when it is still possible to fix them.

It is crucial that sufficient resources are included in the project budget to cover the time and costs of training all members of staff. These include the cost of resources being diverted to training rather than something else (opportunity cost).

In this section we discuss in detail the three main parts of the training process: engagement of staff, identifying training needs and developing a training plan.

Engagement of staff

It is much easier to learn to use a system that you believe is going to be of benefit than one you feel is being forced on you and does not support your clinical goals. Training begins with engaging staff in wanting to use the system. It is not just the straightforward task of teaching staff to click their way through the system.

How one engages staff with the system will depend a lot on the findings during the review of the unit, discussed in Chapter 2. Suggestions include involving staff in the process of choosing the CIS, carrying out surveys and assessing computer literacy skills. To recap the example in Chapter 2, a test of computer literacy that asked people to click on a few boxes and navigate a webpage with the use of the back button had the dual purpose of engaging staff and reassuring them that the task of learning to use a computer was manageable.

Other forms of engagement might be to demonstrate the system in workshops, involve staff in customization, or to ask for their support in developing training materials.

To engage key staff from a range of clinical disciplines is important as they will spread the word to colleagues.

The correct selection of the implementation team will be integral to encouraging staff engagement.

A clinically credible team, recognized within the unit, with good interpersonal skills, will do much to encourage and motivate the staff.

Identifying training needs

Training needs will be identified once the groups to be trained have been decided.

Initial thoughts may be that all staff across all disciplines should be trained in the same way to the same level. However, this may not be the most efficient process.

Nursing staff make up the largest proportion of any critical care workforce and will need training on all aspects of the system. They will have the most hands-on experience of the system on a day-to-day basis once it is in place. Nurses will often be the ones showing the system to other or new users.

Even within the nursing structure though there will be variations in training needs, particularly if one section of nurses has additional responsibilities (e.g. practitioners who have prescribing rights).

Medical staff will not need to learn all aspects of the system – for example, they will not need to know about entering or validating observations, but they will need to know how to read data, enter records and prescribe.

Allied healthcare professionals such as pharmacists and physiotherapists may need training on interpreting and accessing data.

A clear training needs analysis should be put together early in the project, so that a realistic period of training can be formed. An example of a training needs analysis is shown in Table 6.1.

By examining the training needs, it is possible to begin to form an idea of relative training times – for example, nursing staff will require a longer period of training than the secretarial staff.

One group that is often overlooked are people not normally on the unit, but for whom some provision is required. It may be

Table 6.1 Identification of key training areas related to staff groups

	Entering observations	Navigating reading system	Prescribing	Reading/ validating prescriptions	Entering records	Read only
Nursing staff	Yes	Yes		Yes	Yes	
Senior practitioners	Yes	Yes	Yes	Yes	Yes	
Medical staff		Yes	Yes		Yes	
Visiting medical staff						Yes
AHPs		Yes			Yes	
Secretary						Yes

necessary to devise a CIS 'crash course' of as short a duration as possible to equip such staff with the basic skills they need to use the CIS effectively.

Skills gap analysis

A second area to be included within an analysis is the identification of a knowledge/skills gap. Training needs may be two-fold, in computer use and in the CIS itself, and so understanding of the skills gap is crucial.

There may be only a few staff who have previous experience with a CIS, and so the use of the system is likely to be a steep learning curve for most, with nearly all staff requiring similar training.

Computer skills are a different matter and there are a variety of ways to assess the level of computer literacy, from staff questionnaires to basic computer skills tests (as referred to in Chapter 2).

Before any assessment takes place, the basic skills required must be identified. There is no point assessing staff on data entry into an Excel spreadsheet if this is never needed on the system.

Most CIS will only require basic IT skills – management of a mouse, typing and navigating around pages.

Computer literacy may differ between staff groups, and senior doctors may be more reticent about acquiring these skills, seeing them as not relevant or as secretarial work. Computer training must be focused on the needs of each staff group and may need to include a strategy for reluctant people to take part, such as incentives or barring of access to the system to those who have not completed a certain level of training (although this may cause other problems).

Train the trainers

Choosing the group of trainers is key to a successful implementation. The size of the group will depend on the size of the project and how many staff need to be trained.

There are a number of options that could be considered:

1. Use of external trainers, such as the ones provided by the vendor – this has the advantage of using a group of staff who are very familiar with the system and their use as trainers

does not take them away from clinical work within the unit. Disadvantages include that they are not familiar with the clinical work within the unit and will therefore probably be less able to relate the system to the patient's pathway. If the decision is made to use the company training team to train all staff, questions must be asked early in the negotiations about commitment and availability. For all except very small units, there will be a considerable expectation in time needed to cover training requirements.

2. Use of existing unit staff – decisions need to be made about whether this is an existing teaching team or whether you draw from a range of staff. Using staff from the unit has the major advantage of meaning they can teach the system within the clinical setting, embedding all training into clinical practice. The disadvantage is that this will take them away from their 'day job' for a significant amount of time. Support at senior management level is key to allow their release. There will need to be agreement that this is protected released time and cannot be pulled back as a reactive measure against staff shortages. Whether existing teaching staff or a combination is used will probably depend on the numbers required. Few units will have a large enough dedicated teaching team to support the training. Using clinical staff increases credibility and encourages acceptance of the system. As staff trainers will remain on the unit, they can continue to offer support on the unit after the training has finished.

3. A combination of company and clinical staff – it may be that a combined approach is used at certain stages of the

process. For example, the company will need to train the trainers and then may be required at 'go-live' date to provide secondary support to the clinical team.

Within the training team, there needs to be an identified team leader who can motivate and direct the team during the planning and training phases. This does not necessarily need to be the most senior person, although the education lead for the unit is the obvious choice. This role will be key to maintaining the momentum of the training programme as well as providing support to the teaching team – training can be a lonely and arduous task at a time when such a major change is being introduced!

Choosing a team that can work well together, and can support not only the unit staff but each other is an important part of the selection process. Staff who are unsure about the system or fearful of it will often vent their concerns on the trainers – an opportunity to debrief as a group is vital to minimize stress during the training period. This becomes even more important during the implementation phase, when emotions can (and will) run high.

The level that these trainers are trained to needs to be addressed early in the planning. It is probably impractical to train them all as super-users (i.e. able to customize the system) but they do need to have an understanding of the way the system works so that as questions arise during training they can answer them accurately. An understanding of what is and is not possible makes the trainers more credible. The training team need to have a clear understanding of how the CIS will work in practice so that they can devise a training plan that encompasses all the critical points. This is when local knowledge is very important.

Developing a training plan

Once training needs (and trainers) have been identified, a plan can be put in place to carry out the training.

Training people on the CIS is not very different from training them in the use of any other equipment in a critical care unit. This will involve identifying the competencies to be achieved by each staff group, developing appropriate training materials and continuing to refine them for use.

Developing a written training plan covering all aspects is required, especially if there are a number of different trainers delivering the training. A clear plan will ensure there is consistency between sessions.

An important consideration in developing a training plan is to acknowledge the different learning styles which will be met, this means trainers need to be flexible (see Table 6.2).

It is not surprising that it is easier to train people who have no previous experience with paper-based charts than it is to get people to switch from their previous habits around the use of charts to embracing the new possibilities that a CIS presents to them.

How should the training be carried out?

With a training plan in hand, the next step is to decide how long the training should last and when it should start.

Table 6.2 Relating individual learning styles to CIS training

Learning style	Related to CIS training
Auditory	Learns best in a lecture style forum. Likes to listen to instructions. May not respond well to the more informal hands-on style of learning necessary for CIS training.
Visual	Prefers visual stimuli – likes to read handouts and look at images. Will relate well to learning the computer system by looking at its presentation
Tactile	Learns best by doing – these staff will benefit from working their way round the computer screen to see how it works. They will particularly benefit from having an individual computer to 'play' on during training.

Following completion of the skills gap analysis, there should be a clearer idea of how long would be reasonable for training the bulk of staff, although there must be provision within the plan for staff who require extra training.

Differing amounts of time will be allocated to different staff groups depending on what they need to learn and their availability for training. Medical staff are notoriously difficult to arrange formal training with, and they may have to have a more flexible ad-hoc system set up. Formal training as a first introduction to the system for the main user group of nursing staff will probably need to last for several hours for each member of staff – this would allow for a thorough introduction to the system and ensure staff gain confidence in navigating around the various pages.

When to commence training is a critical discussion point for the planning team. Once an implementation date has been chosen, the time to start training can be identified.

If the training is carried out early, over a period of several months before the implementation, it is easier to schedule and puts less of a strain on the unit's staff resources. It has the advantage of garnering interest and commitment to the system. However, staff are likely to forget what they have learnt about system use, particularly if there is any delay in the go-live date, which is more common than one might expect. What has to be expected with early training is that there will need to be significant training repeated around the go-live date.

Conversely, doing training close to the go-live date increases the resource pressure but gives staff an opportunity to put their training into practice quickly. If the unit is large, with a high number of staff requiring training it is difficult to train all the staff in a shorter period of time.

It is better to formally roster staff with study time for this training, rather than trying to take them from within a clinical shift. Formal study time allows plans to ensure that the whole team receive training. Rostering time demonstrates the importance attached to the training and shows support at senior level.

What level of readiness is required for the training system?

This question is particularly relevant for units whose system has been customized, whether by unit staff or by professionals.

It is unlikely that the system will be entirely ready until just before the go-live date. This raises the question of whether the training should be done intensely at the last minute, or whether a more generic version of the system should be used. Taking this latter option gives more flexibility in scheduling the training. It can be done over a wider span of time and will not be affected by delays in the customization process. However, users may complain that they have to 'relearn' the system once the fully customized CIS is in use; they may feel that they have learnt on a system that bears little resemblance to the finished product. This can cause some stress at go-live.

One solution that attempts to minimize disadvantages is early training on a generic system and a large amount of support during the go-live period.

Where should training take place?

A suitable venue has to be found if more than one person will be trained at a time (and to train staff individually would be extremely time consuming and probably less effective). In many hospitals, where training rooms are at a premium, this can be a challenge. Ideally, the room should be block booked for the whole period of training, allowing the team a base to work from.

It is essential that there are sufficient computers in the training room to allow for one per attendee.

Learning is much easier if each person is able to navigate around the system themselves. Sharing facilities tends to lead to the more computer-literate person dominating the session, leading to demoralization of the less confident member.

Timelines

One clear factor from the areas identified in this chapter is that planning before training is essential to ensure success. It is useful to prepare a timeline showing the order in which things should be done, into which the project team can then insert dates.

Use of trainers at implementation

Factored into the time required for training by the trainers is the need for their availability to continue to train and assist staff over the implementation period.

Planning for implementation is included in Chapter 5 and it must be remembered that there will be heavy demands on trainers' time over this period. It is at this point, more than any other, that the cohesiveness of the trainer group will be tested as the implementation period will undoubtedly be a very stressful time for staff working on the unit.

Those who are perceived as responsible (because they are doing all the training) will often bear the brunt of this stress.

Key points

- Planning prior to training is essential for a successful training program.
- Training the trainers is essential.
- Training requires time and resources.

Chapter 7

Customizing a CIS

Introduction

Customization is part of every CIS implementation.

In this chapter the specifics of the customization process will be explained.

The first section looks at the customization primer, discussing the differences that arise in deciding who carries out the customization and when it is done.

The next section presents useful concepts drawn from software engineering to support the customization process. These can be used regardless of whether the actual customization programming is done by a healthcare professional (user-customization) or by IT professionals (standard customization).

Customization primer

What is customization?

Customization is a process that allows an institution to adapt a piece of software, in this case a CIS, to the context and workflow of the unit. The amount of customization possible will depend on the CIS and the vendor.

Table 7.1 Common elements of a CIS that can be customized

What	Examples
Forms for inputting data	Nurses' observations, medical notes
Reports for extracting data	Documentation to be sent to the ward, research report
User interface	Grouping of data, headings
Database	Names and type of data elements stored

Forms and reports are customizable in most CISs. These allow some flexibility in mapping the CIS to the workflow and gaining from the data in the system.

For example, customization can change the fields on data collection forms used by nurses to enter their hourly observations and arrange them in the order normally done in the unit.

Common elements of a CIS that can be customized are listed in Table 7.1.

Adjusting the user-interface and creating a database are larger projects, but give the clinical teams much more control over the use of data in their units.

Who does the customization?

Customization can be done by a range of people or entities.

At one end of the spectrum, customization is done by the vendor who sells the CIS. At the other, customization is done by a select number of healthcare practitioners in the institution in which the CIS will be used.

There are a number of options, including the customization being done by an IT consultancy, by the local IT department, or a mix of IT and healthcare professionals.

The difference is similar to buying a ready-made model aeroplane from a speciality shop, or building one from LEGO® blocks. In the first case, with increasing amounts of money it is possible to buy and have adapted almost any kind of aeroplane, but once complete there are limits to the changes that can be made. In the second case LEGO® provides the building blocks and some instructions, and the blocks can be configured in various ways to match the initial vision. If, in time, it is necessary to change the model that has been built, then the building blocks can be reconfigured.

Buying a system customized by the vendor decreases the amount of work required by the institution to get a CIS implemented and ensures that the system has been properly built and tested, and will be maintained.

The drawback to this approach is that the cost of the customization is likely to be high. The amount of customization needed may be more than estimated. The lead healthcare professional has to figure out how to translate their clinical vision into the system. This can be extremely challenging, and a whole field of research is dedicated to this issue. This can drive up costs beyond expectations. A further issue is the time lag between the requested customization and its delivery.

Carrying out the customization in-house by healthcare practitioners eases problems of cost, translation and time lag.

Disadvantages are that clinical resources need to be diverted to the development of CIS, which can take a substantial amount of time. It requires that there be people in the clinical team interested in learning some extra IT skills and gaining an understanding of basic software engineering concepts.

The less common options, and for most contexts the less helpful, are to have the customization done by IT consultants or the in-house IT department. Vendors have an advantage over IT consultants in that they have knowledge of the system. This gives them the opportunity to charge more. If IT consultants are used, once they have figured out the structure of the system, they too can charge more. Not much is gained. The in-house IT department is not ideal, because IT personnel are usually trained as systems administrators rather than software engineers. Although both of these areas deal with computers, the skills are different.

Who does the customization will depend on the resources of the unit and the extent of the customization. Regardless of who customizes the system, clinical user or professional IT consultant, there will need to be a team who determines what these customizations should look like (e.g. forms). As with all aspects of CIS choice and implementation, a multidisciplinary team is needed to determine the appropriate customization. The diversity of this team ensures that decisions that affect all disciplines are reasonable and that there is expertise for particular forms and reports in each area. Including a variety of people on the customization team will ensure that if a person leaves, the knowledge-base remains.

When to customize

Customization happens in stages. A substantial amount of customization happens before the go-live date. Experience suggests that customization continues for at least two or three months after go-live as the opportunity to interact with the system raises necessary or helpful changes.

Beyond most people's expectations, customization is likely to continue throughout the life of the CIS as staff find ways that it can support improvements in clinical practice, or when clinical practice develops.

It is important to note that customizations before go-live should be tried with the users before the customization process is finished to ensure that there are not mistakes or misunderstandings between staff in the unit and those doing the customization.

This is true for all kinds of customizable systems, even though user-customizable systems can be continually adapted. When considering who customizes, the need for continued customization should be considered.

Useful concepts

The healthcare professionals who carry out customization work are doing some form of software engineering. Although much of the programming may be hidden or done by someone else, the design work is the same.

User-centred design

User-centred design is a standard approach to creating a piece of software that users want to use. It is an iterative cycle of understanding user requirements, generating an appropriate solution and evaluating it against the needs of the user. It is an approach that is useful when designing parts of the CIS, or creating new customizations.

1. Gathering requirements

The first step in creating a customizable element of the CIS is to find out what a particular group needs.

For units transitioning from a paper form system that already supports their work, needs may initially be met by encapsulating the paper forms. New customizations will arise that necessitate requirements gathering.

Staff or disciplines requesting new customizations should be encouraged to write down their needs and perhaps even draw a sketch of what they expect. This will help them define their needs and increase the likelihood that they are consistent and can be interpreted.

Information that will be needed at this stage (depending on the type of customization) will include the following: data, type of data (e.g. number, list, etc.), size of columns for each piece of data, and any details about layout.

Staff may be unfamiliar with data types and what customization tools can do, such as restrictions on the range of numbers inputted. It helps if the person doing the customization asks specific questions concerning the type of each kind of data.

It is useful to ask staff about their choices to see if anything else can be discovered about their needs.

If the project is large, such as creating a database, a space should be dedicated to the project for its duration, so that data elements can be written up on wall charts and grouped or moved around as necessary. This is very common in design and is extremely helpful in increasing the capacity to focus on the needs.

2. Generating a solution

Discussing a solution in the abstract can lead to miscommunication.

It is useful for the customizer to show the requester a quick sketch as an interpretation of their needs. For example, if the requester proposes a report about the number of bed days, then the customizer shows them what the CIS is likely to produce.

Concrete representations of ideas, such as sketches, provide a good discussion tool to ensure that both customizer and requester have a shared idea. This process can help eliminate miscommunication before the customization is done and help the requester further develop their ideas.

It is a recognized problem in software engineering that people rarely know what they want before they have it and, at that point, it is too late!

3. Evaluating the solution

It is important to evaluate, even informally, the solution in practice.

It is not uncommon that when tried in practice it is discovered that elements do not work and new ideas spring up.

Evaluation can be done for simple customizations by walking through a sketch in the environment in which it will be used. For example, a sketch of a new nursing form can be used by a single nurse at the bedside as a trial.

If the customizations are done on a user-customizable system then changes can be easily made. If the customizations are done by IT professionals then changes will be difficult and expensive. It is therefore essential that the solution is tried before it is customized into the CIS.

Documentation

Documentation is one of the most important, albeit laborious, parts of software engineering. If the customization is done by IT professionals, it can be expected that documentation will be done as part of their professional practice. It is worthwhile requesting that the documentation be included in the contract. This will avoid potential problems if further customization is carried out by a different IT consultancy.

If the system is user-customizable, documenting will be an important part of the customization work. Documenting refers to explanations of how each customization has been done and giving reasons for particular choices. For example, there are multiple data types that can be assigned to a data element and they can be combined in various ways. The choice of which one was used should be documented to make it possible to change this decision in the future without causing knock-on effects to other parts of the customization.

Documentation provides a starting point for any new customizer working on the system.

Documentation tools are standard in professional software engineering packages, but may not be available in user-customization tools.

It is adequate to keep a log of customizations and rationales in a text document. For those who have a highly customized system, a chart of how all the pages fit together and documentation of which data types are on which pages will make it easier to navigate the system as it grows and will help in testing and integration.

Testing and integration

Testing and integration can be expected from IT professionals who are carrying out customization work.

With a user-customizable CIS, these jobs will fall to the health professional, perhaps unknowingly, and are crucial to avoid hiccups in the functioning of the CIS.

Once a new customization has been done, it is best to upload it to a test environment to ensure that it does not cause problems for the main CIS system. User-customizable systems should separate the functioning of the CIS and customizable elements, but it is always best to check. Testing will show whether the customized element is working as expected before staff are directed to use it.

Integration is perhaps more challenging than testing. It refers to changing an old customization for a new one while the system is live.

Ideally, the customization tools should facilitate this, but often they do not. If an integration tool is not provided, use of a particular aspect of the system (e.g. form or report) needs to be stopped, while the new one is put in place. There can be lengthy delays if this is the case.

Box 7.1

On one unit, changes needed to be made to the pressure ulcer record page, but each time this was tried, the form was in use, meaning the update could not happen.

Coordinating all staff on a large and busy critical care unit to stop using a form at the same time is challenging. It is worthwhile asking the vendor about how integration is done and how it might be facilitated by their tools.

Version control

Version control is a useful software engineering practice that reduces mistakes.

Each time a customization is worked on, it should be saved as a new version. Some people use a number system, for example medical_notes_v1, medical_notes_v2. Others use the date.

If there are several people working on a customization, the initials of the person working on the latest version can support collaboration and ensure that other people's work is not lost.

If it is difficult to change the buttons to the new file name, old versions can be saved with negative numbers, with 0 always being the current one.

Poor version control means that work can be accidentally deleted. Previous versions provide a back-up in case a recent customization does not work as expected and alters the system inappropriately.

Box 7.2

One customizer found an option in a user-customizable CIS that allowed her to share an algorithm between pages. Only when it was too late did she discover that she could not 'un-share' the algorithm to modify it in each form.

Version control allows one to return to an old version and bypass problems.

Hidden dependencies

Testing and version control are particularly helpful for healthcare professionals who are customizing because computer programming languages will contain hidden dependencies.

Some commands will have multiple behaviours that are linked and change the system in unexpected ways.

For example, if an algorithm is re-used in numerous parts of the program and then subsequently changed, it will change in all places and not just where changed.

IT professionals are often aware where hidden dependencies might be found, but healthcare professionals may not be. Good version control can make mistakes easy to recover from.

Box 7.3

Using a specific CIS, the customizer can construct a database query in a query tool provided with the CIS and then insert the results into a report either by cutting and pasting it or by linking it. If the customizer chooses the latter (linking), and somebody changes the query in the query tool, it will change in the report without notice. Changing the query after having used the former option (copy and paste) will not have this behaviour and the result in the report will remain as per the original formula.

Debugging

Computer programs rarely work at the first attempt, even when created by very experienced professionals.

The programmer then enters a state of debugging, in order to find the problem.

Debugging strategies usually mean changing small bits of the code to isolate the problem so that it can be fixed. Customizers of user-customizable systems should expect to do a substantial amount of debugging.

It is not a measure of competence, but part of the process.

Gardeners

Every organization that carries out some kind of user-customization will find someone who is particularly keen to work with the IT system and is savvy in getting it to be even more useful.

This person has been termed the gardener in computer science literature, because they constantly 'tend and grow' the capabilities of the IT system.

This person is not an IT specialist, but a person with domain knowledge who has 'figured out' productive ways to use the IT system.

Gardeners are invaluable to organizations because of their domain knowledge. They need support to continue to innovate. Organizations who find ways to recognize customization achievements and give the gardeners appropriate time for customizing usually gain the most.

Professional IT experience may need to be made available to the gardeners to increase their skills and ensure that technological details have been attended to, such as the need for solutions to work on multiple types of computers. IT professionals on their own can rarely propose innovative uses of technology in a particular domain as they are not domain experts.

Usability

A CIS requires good usability to be user-friendly.

Good usability is a term used in technology communities to denote aspects of a piece of software that support a user's cognition.

Table 7.2 Assessing usability of CIS

What	Examples
Visibility of system status	The system should always keep users informed about what is going on, through appropriate feedback within a reasonable time.
Consistency and standards	Users should not have to wonder whether different words, situations, or actions mean the same thing. Follow conventions.
Error prevention	Even better than good error messages is a careful design which prevents a problem from occurring. Either eliminate error-prone conditions or check for them and present users with a confirmation option before they commit to the action.
Recognition rather than recall	Minimize the user's memory load by making objects, actions and options visible. The user should not have to remember information from one part of the dialogue to another. Instructions for use of the system should be visible or easily retrievable whenever appropriate.
Aesthetic and minimalist design	Dialogues should not contain information which is irrelevant or rarely needed. Every extra unit of information in a dialogue competes with the relevant units of information and diminishes their relative visibility

Usability studies are common practice in the development of software in most domains, but less often used or demanded in healthcare settings. Such studies look at the ease of carrying out common tasks in a piece of software. If a system is customized by a vendor, such tests should be insisted upon.

Useful guidelines have been drawn from Jakob Nielson's ten usability heuristics and are listed in Table 7.2. These are applicable if the system is user-customizable.

A much larger number of techniques for assessing the usability of a CIS can be found in the literature, such as in Saleem *et al.* (2009).

Customization tips

It is the healthcare professionals who need to translate the clinical vision into the CIS through the design of the forms, reports, or other customizable elements, regardless of who carries out the customization.

This section gives a number of general tips from the authors' and editor's experience.

The power game

Most CISs offer ways to constrain the user to carry out tasks in certain ways.

One common example of this is required fields. In other words, the user cannot save the data without filling in the required fields, something people will be familiar with from website registrations.

Making too many requirements can cause healthcare practitioners to misuse the system, filling in dots or zeros to boxes that they do not want to fill in, or clicking checklists without doing them, in order to get on to a different part of the system. Not only does this not achieve the purpose of the required fields, it frustrates the healthcare practitioners, and corrupts the database.

It is recommended that required fields be limited to data elements that are absolutely necessary.

The power game that can be played through the CIS is more explicit with alerts.

Alerts are messages that pop-up to remind or instruct a healthcare professional about the action that they are carrying out. It is difficult to customize alerts so that they are always relevant and not inappropriately frequent.

It is not uncommon to have alert fatigue, which causes people to ignore all alerts, even potentially significant ones, such as an allergy conflict with a medication. Alerts can threaten the identity of the healthcare professionals, leading to subversive behaviour.

Box 7.4

One hospital's guidelines for a specific drug allowed dosages of up to 10 mg to be prescribed. Experience in the critical care unit in this hospital was that dosages above 5 mg caused patients to bleed. In response, the CIS was customized so that a warning sign flashed on the screen, stating the safe limit of 5 mg and asking whether the prescriber really wanted to give more. In reaction, two consultants consistently prescribed 6 mg as a way of indicating their dissatisfaction with the message on the CIS. This could put patients at risk and is therefore not a situation that the CIS should inspire.

Encouraging good clinical practice

There are other, less coercive, means of encouraging good clinical practice through thoughtful design of the CIS.

A very basic, but important, rule of thumb is to always put buttons where people expect them to be. While this may seem obvious, it takes care to do, and design professionals often spend hours correcting mistakes when doing an expert review.

To do this, one needs to be very aware of the work practices of the people using the system. A healthcare professional in one discipline may not be as familiar with practices in another. The example in box 7.5 below shows how powerful this simple rule can be.

Box 7.5

Patients who have had a specific device inserted require that their dressings are checked every hour. This was included in a checklist of patients of this type in a CIS. As the checklist was not mandatory and it was not in an expected place, it was overlooked. Nurses for a recent patient had not checked the dressings in 36 hours and the patient was found to be without an appropriate dressing for this period of time. The solution of this problem was to move the checklist to a place that the nurse might expect to click on it.

Another customization tip that can encourage good practice is to make good practice easy. A good example of this is to make protocol drugs easy to access and the order form pre-filled, while making the prescription of non-protocol drugs time-consuming.

User-customization tips

For those institutions that have healthcare practitioners do the customization, there are a few more issues that need to be considered, namely starting points and vendor assessment.

Starting points

There are a number of different starting points for such systems.

Some institutions like to start from scratch, building their own databases and all their forms. This requires real dedication from the leads and there is the possibility that mistakes will be made, even though the vendor should provide guidance.

Another option is to work with a template from another institution. This decreases the amount of work to be done and creates a starting point for those who may feel overwhelmed by the process. The disadvantage is that the institution has to live with the mistakes of the institution from which the template is borrowed.

In some cases, a third option may be to use a template supplied by the vendor. This will probably have fewer mistakes and may be easier for the vendor to update over time, but it may be costly and not have the clinical vision embedded in a system created by other clinicians.

Vendor assessment

If a unit is customizing its own CIS, the vendor relationship is crucial. Ensure that the vendor is prepared to support training and has the resources to do so. Examine the initial training offered as well as continuing training and costs. The support materials, such as training manuals and documentation, need to be considered.

Be aware that training may be a source of income for CIS providers and consider whether the costs will be manageable within the set budget. It is not possible to customize a CIS and maintain it without training and support.

Another issue that may be raised is that of liability. Investigate what liability the vendor holds. They may have designed their product in such a way that they are not liable for any mistakes that come from poor or untested customization.

Although an institution can take steps, as described in the section on 'Useful concepts', to ensure that problems do not arise, it is important to be clear on these issues before a legal case raises them.

Vendor conflicts

Buying a user-customizable system requires some initiative on the part of the organization to get the most from the system.

Research has highlighted that significant customization is not necessarily in the interest of the vendor. The more a system is customized, the more resource-intensive it is for the vendor to upgrade the system, but the more the organization can integrate the system into their practices.

This tension needs to be actively managed by an organization that has any level of customization of its system. Careful attention should be paid to the maintenance contract of such a system.

Key points

- A range of customizable systems are available, and choices need to be made about who customizes and plans made about when it is done.
- Regardless of who carries out the customization the clinical vision and its translation into the CIS needs to be done by the healthcare practitioners in the institution.

TO LEARN MORE

J. J. Saleem, A. L. Russ, P. Sanderson, T. R. Johnson, J. Zhang, D. F. Sittig, 2009. Current challenges and opportunities for better integration of human factors research with development of clinical information systems purpose: informatics and patient safety. *IMIA Yearbook of Medical Informatics 2009*: 48–58.

Chapter 8

Leadership

Introduction

Strong leadership has a key role in achieving successful implementation of a CIS.

This chapter describes what constitutes effective leadership of a CIS implementation, beginning with a discussion of clinical leadership and how to build a team.

The next section examines how the team can maintain staff morale by understanding how to provide support throughout the process of change. As success ultimately comes from meeting the goals of the CIS, how to lessen the disparity between objectives and outcomes and how to track costs and benefits in practice is discussed.

Clinical leadership

A CIS introduced into a single unit is likely to be instigated by clinical staff who will continue to play a significant role in its development.

When a CIS is implemented across an organization, it is not uncommon for the decision to have been made by management, and the task of implementing to fall to the hospital IT department, with or without the assistance of external consultants.

If this is the case, it is essential that substantial clinical buy-in and leadership is generated for the project. How this can be done is discussed in the next section. If clinical leadership cannot be garnered, it is worth questioning whether a CIS is the right choice.

Research has demonstrated that even a well-designed CIS can fail if the clinical staff refuse to embrace it.

Clinical leadership may be drawn from any of the clinical disciplines. It is not uncommon for implementation to be guided by senior nursing staff, for example. If only one discipline leads the implementation there is always the question of whether the other disciplines will follow, particularly the doctors. Clinical leadership should include staff from the multidisciplinary team. This ensures all perspectives are represented and support is drawn from all clinical disciplines.

The clinical leadership team may vary in size, but should be large enough to be robust if people leave the institution, and be able to represent all the units involved in the implementation.

Building the team

Roles

The three main roles that need to be filled in a clinical leadership team for a CIS implementation project are shown in Table 8.1.

Table 8.1 The three main roles in a clinical leadership team

Figurehead	A well-respected, often senior, member of the clinical community who acts as an advocate and spokesperson for CIS.
	Usually not directly involved with its implementation. They need to be a visibly active user.
Clinical lead	Acts as an advocate and spokesperson for the CIS, but actively manages the overall implementation process, taking on responsibilities such as chairing the steering group, and guiding system design, although typically without getting involved in the development.
Clinical project teams	Hands-on people, who are not only advocates for the CIS, but also manage the implementation process on a day-to-day level.
	Likely to be actively involved in the design, development and customization of the system.

In bringing together the multidisciplinary clinical leadership team it is important to include a range of people from across disciplines, as appropriate.

For example, there should be a clinical lead and several project team members from the medical, nursing and allied health professions, but there are likely to be just one or two figureheads.

As noted in Chapter 2, it is essential to build this team from the inception of the idea of a CIS as it will take time and effort.

Characteristics

The members of the clinical team may be selected because of their role, but the team also needs to have a balance of the following characteristics: influence, vision, authority and credibility (Figure 8.1).

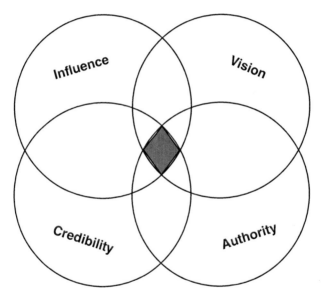

Figure 8.1

Influence provides the ability to obtain and direct resources as necessary (and appropriate) to the CIS implementation project.

Vision provides direction to keep the customization of the CIS on track to support clinical work.

Authority, especially if associated with a senior organizational role, provides the ability to influence and, if necessary, mandate changes in work practices that will be associated with the introduction of the CIS.

Credibility provides evidence that clinicians' concerns are suitably represented in system design and demonstrates to peers that the CIS is working well.

It is unlikely that each person in the clinical leadership team will have all of these characteristics, although they may have several. Forming a strong leadership team is about obtaining a good balance of these characteristics across the team.

Potential problems

A strong clinical leadership team often requires senior clinical staff diverting their attention from other projects.

As discussed in Chapter 2, clinical time will need to be allocated to the implementation of a CIS and this should be considered when choosing a system and planning implementation. Some of the demands on senior clinical time can be reduced by taking a team approach.

A further advantage of a team, as opposed to an individual, is that it avoids the problem of the credibility of the system being affected by an individual's reputation, involving the CIS in organizational politics.

A team provides a stable structure to continue with the project in the event of one person leaving. Careful construction of the clinical leadership team will help to minimize problems.

Maintaining staff morale

Introduction of a CIS will affect staff morale.

The clinical leadership team should monitor staff morale throughout implementation and take steps to maintain it.

Proactive strategies are needed, such as communication and formal methods of monitoring staff morale. Being aware of problems and actively reaching out to those who struggle to adjust to the CIS is a crucial part of leading the implementation to success.

Common anxieties

The CIS is likely to engender anxieties in many of the clinical staff regardless of their speciality, age or experience. Some of this may come from fear of computers, which can be addressed through preparatory exercises as described in Chapter 2.

Much of the anxiety is due to the more general fear of change. A CIS will replace familiar work practices with new tasks. This requires people to make a large effort in adjusting their work practice. While doing this, they may question their identity within the organization, their ability to carry out the new tasks, as well as the possible loss of status if they are seen as struggling to use the CIS.

Some may also question the security of their jobs. Although many of these worries may be hypothetical, positive

Table 8.2 The four stages of responses to organizational change

Shock
Defensive retreat
Acknowledgement
Acceptance and adaptation

encouragement and good communication are likely to ease the process.

These anxieties should never be underestimated – in one centre, senior staff who had worked within a critical care unit for many years (and were very skilled in their work) found the first few days with the CIS left them feeling like new staff, and made them question their ability to do any of their normal daily roles.

Psychology of change

Responses to organizational change are generally recognized as going through four stages as listed in Table 8.2.

In the first stage, individuals see the impending change as a threat and may even deny that it is happening. They experience fear and uncertainty about the future, causing morale and productivity to fall.

Negative attitudes to the change are strengthened in the second stage as individuals seek to hold on to old practices and challenge new ones. As they recognize that change cannot be avoided, individuals are no longer able to deny it and begin to adjust to the new situation. As they accumulate positive experiences, their confidence grows and they move towards acceptance.

Over time they may come to appreciate the benefits of change and to evaluate the process favourably, sometimes to the extent of directly contradicting their earlier objections.

Recognizing which stage most of the people are in, or perhaps just one particularly troublesome person is in, can help in determining what actions are likely to be most productive. If someone is in shock, for example, it may be best to give them a lighter workload, but if someone has acknowledged that change has happened, positive encouragement for steps of adaption is likely to speed the process.

Recognizing these stages is helpful as a starting point to think about appropriate leadership actions for the whole unit, but it is also important to recognize that people respond to change differently.

These responses to change may be separated into three broad types:

1. Conservers prefer change that maintains the current structure, and may experience stress even at the prospect of change. They value predictability and are often detail focused. Good strategies to work with these people are to establish a clear path of change in a series of small steps to enable them to adjust progressively the range of activities that they feel comfortable with. It can be important to

maintain links back to earlier practices (e.g. showing how the CIS matches what they are familiar with from paper records) and to visibly maintain old practices as a back-up until they are confident with the new systems, such as keeping paper records in a known location.

2. Pragmatists prefer change that produces workable outcomes. They value consultation and focus more on results than structure. They tend to be team oriented and will be willing to adjust to change if it is seen to have general support. Listening to their opinions about the CIS and communicating results is likely to encourage them through the change process.

3. Originators prefer change that challenges current structures. They enjoy risk and uncertainty and tend to be focused on a vision, but may not be excessively concerned about details or practicalities. They are most likely to embrace change associated with a strong clinical vision. Such individuals can be encouraged by being given opportunities to experiment (perhaps in areas that are not critical to core work practices). The challenge for the leadership team is to harness their enthusiasm while ensuring that it is directed in productive ways.

These profiles are helpful in identifying how to interact with specific people throughout the implementation process.

The leadership team will need to be aware that their attitudes to change may not be shared by colleagues.

Some resistance to change is inevitable.

Change usually creates winners and losers – those whose strengths are utilized by the changes and those whose strengths are no longer utilized. Those who feel that they will lose may seek to slow or prevent change. They may do so passively by not changing the way they work. For example, a senior clinician who does not want to use a keyboard may insist that a junior does the typing for them.

Resistance can also be active, creating an oppositional or subversive force. Opposition is a direct challenge to the CIS and can be countered in a number of ways: (1) evidence that questions the claims of opponents, or supports claims of proponents (although this may not always be accepted), (2) strategy (finding ways to divert or weaken opposition), or (3) negotiation.

It is generally best to avoid enforcing change without addressing opponents' concerns, as this is likely to encourage resentment and subversion.

Subversive resistance is more indirect and may involve efforts to 'sabotage' the system, for example by identifying weaknesses in the CIS and focusing attention on them.

Subversion may be difficult to counter as it may be covert and may be denied if detected. If identified, it is important to engage with those involved, rather than to confront them, by identifying their concerns and exploring how they can be addressed.

The clinical leadership team can take the responsibility for managing resistance.

A first step is identifying people who have something to lose from the implementation of the CIS, or may perceive they have something to lose.

For example, senior nurses who do not know how to use a computer may feel that a CIS undermines their authority.

Understanding their reasons for concern and seeing how these concerns can be addressed will go a long way – in this example, through targeted training that acknowledges and does not belittle these concerns. Anticipate what their response is likely to be when help is given and provide incentives for accepting the support.

Although resistance can come from a desire not to change, it is often natural and rational. When people resist, consider carefully what their complaints are about. For example, they may be highlighting unanticipated consequences, the failure of the change initiative to pay attention to significant issues, or wider organizational tensions. Resistance can also be a mechanism for pointing out problems, and these should not be ignored.

Communication

A primary strategy in reducing anxiety and stress preceding implementation of a CIS is to have a functional communication strategy.

Frequent communication keeps people aware of the project's progress, maintains awareness of the project and reminds people that CIS will be going live.

Communication works best when done through a variety of media as people may need to see it more than once or may only attend to certain media. These might include regular newsletters, either printed or through email, a regularly updated website, and meetings, either CIS specific or an agenda item at a general meeting.

Table 8.3 Messages to be communicated to the wider team

Why CIS is being introduced and what the expected benefits are

What CIS will change (and what it won't)

Potential problems/downsides

Criteria for success

Openness to feedback

Any problems that arise

A non-exhaustive list of messages to be communicated is shown in Table 8.3.

People are more likely to accept change if they know why it is being done and how it will help them. It is important to be honest and accurate to set people's expectations appropriately. The CIS will have drawbacks as well as benefits and these need to be communicated.

If people are told the criteria for success, and when these have/ have not been met, they may find it easier to accept the changes. Openness towards feedback often reassures people that they will be listened to if things go badly wrong, providing a safety net so to speak.

Finally, be open about delays and problems. Covering them up will only make their eventual arrival unexpected and therefore more damaging to project credibility. The absence of formal communication will not stop information about the project spreading, so it is better if news, good or bad, is shared promptly and accurately through 'official channels'.

Monitoring morale

Morale can be monitored both formally and informally. Surveys that ask questions about job satisfaction are one formal way.

With preparation, a survey can be given before implementation and then four and twelve months after implementation to ensure that staff morale does not dip over a long period of time.

Proxy measures, such as absenteeism, staff turnover and volume of comments in the feedback system (if in place), can also give an indication of the trends in staff morale.

Informal feedback may also be useful if it comes from trusted sources. Informal mechanisms might be the most useful in determining appropriate solutions.

It is to be expected that staff morale will dip after such a major change as the implementation of a CIS, but it is important to monitor it to ensure that this dip does not become permanent and that staff concerns are attended to.

There are several free existing evaluation tools that can be used to monitor staff morale. The CIS evaluation tool (http://cisevaluation.com) provides a pre- and post-survey and scoring guide. It is perhaps the easiest to administer.

Leading to success

Objectives versus outcomes

A successful implementation will not be the same in all places, but will depend on whether the outcomes meet the local objectives.

As emphasized in Chapter 3, if these objectives are realistic and honest, it is more likely that they will be met and that people will perceive the CIS as a success.

Objectives can be progressively stepped up as people adjust to the changes. A first goal for example may be to introduce a CIS that looks like the former paper-based system. After a period of adjustment, the goal may be to change problematic work practices. This staged approach helps people adjust to the ideas as they come, rather than forcing too much change at once.

Significant change at the beginning may result in revolt and the failure of the implementation. The longer that the CIS is used, the less likely it is that there will be calls for a return to the old system, and therefore the more opportunity there will be to continue to develop work practices and the development of the CIS in support of them.

One issue to be aware of is that the CIS is likely to highlight underlying problems in clinical work practices.

This happens because the previous work-arounds will no longer be possible, pushing the problem into the limelight. For example, if clinicians did not write-up patient discharge summaries before the CIS was introduced, they are not likely to do so afterwards, but the system will make it more apparent as it will indicate if these have not been completed.

It is important to emphasize to those who highlight a problem that it is not caused by the CIS, but is a long-standing issue in the unit that the CIS has simply made visible. If this is not done, the CIS will be blamed for everything that happens and it will not be regarded as successful.

Costs and benefits

The business plan created to get approval for the system will undoubtedly have a cost–benefit discussion or even calculation.

In practice it is very difficult to measure costs and benefits and it may not be possible to see any benefit at the unit level.

Time savings gained in one area will often be spent in another. The CIS may also change practices so substantially that it is difficult to compare with the paper-based system. Quantitative benefits may be shown at the institutional level and at the clinical level, encouraging staff to use and continue to support the system.

Key points

- Leading a successful implementation of a CIS starts with building the appropriate clinical leadership team.
- The team needs to be multidisciplinary, with members who can take on all of the roles required and possess a mix of the essential characteristics.
- The team needs to take responsibility for monitoring and supporting staff morale and ensuring that the objectives are appropriately set and communicated.
- The team should keep in mind what benefits are realistic to measure and how that might affect objectives setting.

TO LEARN MORE

C. E. Aydin, 2005. Survey methods for assessing social impacts of computers in healthcare organizations. In J. G. Anderson and C. E. Aydin (eds), *Evaluating the Organizational Impact of Healthcare Information Systems – Health Informatics*, 2nd edn. New York: Springer, pp. 75–128.

Chapter 9

Impact on clinical workflow

Introduction

The first eight chapters of this book have given practical guidance on choosing and implementing a CIS. In this chapter, the focus is on the impact a CIS can have on clinical practice once in place, and, in particular, on adoption patterns, potential improvements in practices, and changes in workflow. Where possible, evidence is presented from published research studies to support the arguments made.

Adoption patterns

A CIS is only effective if people use it.

Research evidence indicates that adoption can be mixed, even in units or hospitals in which a CIS has been fully implemented.

Healthcare professionals in these environments may use the system where this is mandated, but may not utilize the full extent of its capabilities, preferring to rely on previous methods or paper.

This leads to inefficiencies as duplicate systems are maintained and creates the potential for errors where there are discrepancies between multiple systems.

Box 9.1

Research evidence

A survey of doctors' use of electronic medical record systems in
32 units in 19 Norwegian hospitals found that only between two and
seven of the 15 tasks supported by the systems were used by doctors,
mainly those associated with reading patient data.

H. Laerum, G. Ellingsen and A. Faxvaag, 2001. Doctors' use of
electronic patient records systems in hospitals: cross sectional
survey, *British Medical Journal* 323(7325): 1344–8.

Willingness to use a CIS is often considered to vary between
different staff groups. A common distinction is made between
nurses and doctors.

Nurses

Nurses are sometimes considered to be a difficult group
to get to adopt a CIS, because they may prioritize patient
care over what is perceived to be administration work. They
may lack computer literacy or be reluctant to change
routines.

A number of studies have shown that nurses, especially in
critical care, often adapt well to CIS. This is said to be because
they already work with a large amount of technology with a
digital interface, such as ventilators and infusion pumps, and
do not make a distinction between this equipment and
information technology.

If the nurses feel that a piece of technology will help them
care for their patients, they are likely to use it.

Box 9.2

Research evidence

Studies of nurses' attitudes to CIS use found mainly positive perceptions. Nurses hoped to have, or were pleased by, less time spent documenting and more time with their patients. Concerns were around reliability. In one study, nursing staff recruitment and retention improved after CIS implementation.

P. Norrie, 2003. What do critical care nurses want from clinical information systems? *Information Technology in Nursing* 15(4): 10–15.

P. Norrie, 2004. A qualitative comparison between critical care sites which use a computerised information system and conventional data management. *Information Technology in Nursing* 16(2): 5–9.

D. J. Fraenkel, M. Cowie and P. Daley, 2003. Quality benefits of an intensive care clinical information system. *Critical Care Medicine* 31(1): 120–5.

This suggests that the adoption of a CIS by nurses is likely to be successful if a clear case is made to show how it will support care for their patients.

Authority relationships within hospitals mean that nurses may consider that they are expected to comply with instructions from senior figures and may not, overtly, resist CIS use if this is mandated. The problem is that passive resistance and lack of motivation to use a CIS, where this is imposed, may mean that the system is rarely used to its full potential. Compliance with mandated use cannot therefore be considered as reliable evidence of acceptance.

Medical staff

Adoption rates among medical staff can vary substantially.

While many of the strongest proponents of CIS use (and often those most active in CIS implementation programmes) are medical staff, a significant minority of medical staff may be actively hostile to CIS adoption.

This may reflect low levels of computer literacy (and consequent concerns about loss of status if CIS use becomes obligatory); organizational politics, where the CIS is associated with a particular specialism or department; long experience of, and investment in, existing systems that the CIS may replace; and differences of opinion regarding the merits of CIS use.

Senior medical staff are likely to be able to avoid CIS use, either by deputizing use to junior colleagues or by ignoring efforts to require them to use it (as there are likely to be few effective sanctions against non-compliance).

Junior doctors, in contrast, typically have few problems with CIS use. Most are computer literate, are expected to do a lot of data entry as part of their job, can be ordered to enter data for senior colleagues and may be less strongly aligned with particular specialisms/departments and so less concerned about, or susceptible to, organizational politics.

Social influence can have a significant effect on adoption.

Friends' positive attitudes towards CIS use, even if they do not necessarily work in the same unit, may encourage individual adoption, although the effect can work in the other direction too, with friends' poor experience of, or attitudes to,

CIS use deterring adoption. Contrary to popular belief, studies have not shown age to be a determining factor.

Box 9.3
Research evidence
Social network analysis of doctors using a CIS in a primary care setting identified that the most likely predictor of adoption was whether friends had adopted. Clinical colleague networks and influence networks were not predictors of adoption.

K. Zheng, R. Padman, D. Krackhardt, M. P. Johnson and H. S. Diamond, 2010. Social networks and physician adoption of electronic health records: insights from an empirical study. *Journal of the American Medical Informatics Association* 17(3): 328–36.
    H. Laerum, G. Ellingsen and A. Faxvaag, 2001. Doctors' use of electronic patient records systems in hospitals: cross sectional survey, *British Medical Journal* 323(7325): 1344–8.

Improvements in clinical practice

The main benefits that are expected from implementation of a CIS are generally considered to be improvements in clinical practice.

E-prescribing and medical ordering

A reduction in adverse drug events as a result of computerized physician order entry (CPOE) is widely identified as one of the key clinical benefits of CIS implementation.

The 2000 US Institute of Medicine report focused on this issue, *To Err is Human: Building a Safety Health System,* has been influential in establishing the case for CIS adoption.

Other studies have identified the potential for computerized physician order entry to introduce new errors. While CPOE is seen as increasing patient safety it should not be considered a panacea.

Box 9.4

Research evidence

A summary of the literature in critical care notes that e-prescribing offers advantages such as legible orders, faster order completion, inventory management and automatic billing. The greatest benefits are realized when the CIS has features to prevent medication errors and adverse drug events. But if e-prescribing is not done carefully, adverse drug events can be facilitated.

D. M. Maslove, N. Rizk and H. J. Lowe, 2011. Computerized physician order entry in the critical care environment: a review of current *literature, Journal of Intensive Care Medicine* 26(3): 165–71.

K. Colpaert and J. Decruyenaere, 2009. Computerized physician order entry in critical care, *Best Practice & Research Clinical Anaesthesiology* 23(1): 27–38.

Box 9.5

Research evidence

A study comparing the quality of handwritten versus computerized prescriptions in a tertiary 25-bedded cardiothoracic intensive care unit found that only 3% of handwritten charts analysed had all immediate administration (STAT) drugs prescribed correctly. Errors included omission of route (8%), date of prescription (8%) and time to be given (25%), and 12% had no dose or an incorrect dose prescribed. All errors of completeness were abolished following CIS implementation and led to a significant improvement in prescribing safety, in a clinical area previously highlighted as having a high rate of adverse drug errors. Legibility, completeness and traceability were no longer possible sources of medication errors.

J. Ali, L. Barrow and A. Vuylsteke, 2010. The impact of computerized physician order entry on prescribing practices in a cardiothoracic intensive care unit. *Anaesthesia* 65(2): 119–23.

Box 9.6
Research evidence
A qualitative and quantitative study of use of a CPOE in a tertiary teaching hospital identified 22 types of error risk. Three-quarters of staff reported observing each of the risks, suggesting that they occurred at least weekly. Examples of potential errors included fragmented CPOE displays preventing a coherent view of patients' medications, antibiotic renewal notices being placed on paper charts rather than in the CPOE system, separation of functions facilitating double dosing and incompatible orders, and inflexible ordering formats generating wrong orders.

R. Koppel, J. P. Metlay, A. Cohen *et al.*, 2005. Role of computerized physician order entry systems in facilitating medication errors, *JAMA* 293: 1197–203.

Documentation

CIS provides legible and often complete patient documentation (Figure 9.1).

Electronic documentation has the advantage of all information being in one place, removing the need to keep track of multiple data sources.

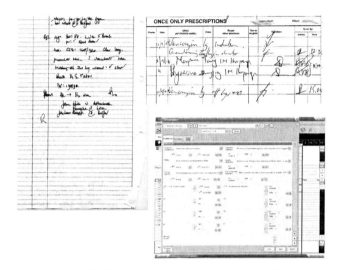

Figure 9.1 Handwritten instructions or summaries can be indecipherable.

Historical documentation is highly accessible and it is less likely to have lost or missing records or data, although IT malfunctions can make this possible.

Electronic documentation can highlight poor data entry, individually or collectively.

The existence of a comprehensive record in which all actions are associated with a particular individual's username can create some anxieties about surveillance and the possibility for retrospective analysis.

Some users may complain that they feel like 'Big Brother' is watching them and this may provoke negative attitudes towards the CIS.

Accountability must be approached sensitively and positively, highlighting people's achievements.

CIS has the potential to provide access to records from any location. This can support allied health professionals, such as pharmacists, consulting the record from their base anywhere in the hospital without needing to visit the ward. It may be useful as a reference point for consultants when they are asked questions when they are not at the bedside. It enables simultaneous access of a record for different disciplines whose jobs may not overlap.

Remote access needs to be done with some caution, as a CIS does not handle all communication, for example updating bedside nurses about prescription changes.

A CIS standardizes the types of data and the formats in which data are recorded. This often means that there is less flexibility for the healthcare professional in describing a patient's condition. In particular, the narrative that some people are particularly drawn to, and that some find particularly informative, may disappear (although staff can exhibit considerable ingenuity in finding ways to reinstate it where it is discouraged).

Some staff may find it very difficult to adapt to a system where they are not able to write a large amount of free text, as the writing process often supports the thinking process.

Data

A CIS can offer completely new ways of using data in clinical practice.

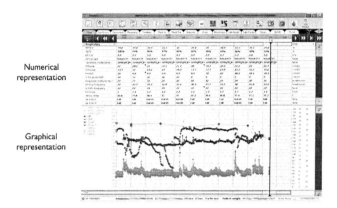

Numerical representation

Graphical representation

Figure 9.2 Data can be reviewed numerically or graphically.

With paper records, all healthcare professionals see the data in the same way. Electronic records allow different representations of data for each professional discipline. For example, a dietician may be mainly interested in data specific to the diet and fluid balance of the patient and only need the data to prescribe feed. A dietician's view of the system can focus on these elements with all other data accessible on an as-needed basis.

Another advantage of CIS is that data can be viewed either numerically or graphically. Graphical data is particularly useful for revealing trends (Figure 9.2).

Care bundle and guideline compliance

Many managers are interested in a CIS because it provides mechanisms with which to encourage, or even enforce, protocols and good practice.

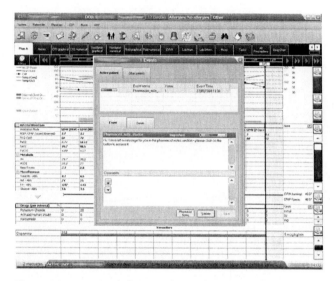

Figure 9.3 Automated alerts can be used to attract clinician attention.

Pop-up reminders can request clinicians to complete required tasks, or the system may not allow data on a page to be saved into the record unless all fields have been filled in (Figure 9.3).

While there is evidence that computerization of guidelines, per se, can increase compliance, such an outcome cannot be guaranteed. Low compliance may not reflect a reluctance to follow care bundles, but rather problems of multi-professional teamworking. For example, completion of all elements of a care bundle may involve medical prescribing and may therefore be delayed until a doctor is available, even if nursing

staff have followed all other procedures in a timely
fashion.

While a CIS can encourage good practice, the technology in
itself is not the answer. A thoughtful, organizational change
approach to the problem is still necessary.

Box 9.7

Research evidence

The introduction of a CIS in a large cardiothoracic CCU improved
compliance with the ventilator care bundle by 6.8%, but the addition
of electronic prompts did not have any further impact upon overall
compliance. Total compliance was only achieved in the single
element actionable at the bedside by the nurse to whom the
electronic prompts were addressed.

A. Ashworth, J. Armstrong, S. T. Webb and A. Vuylsteke, 2009. A
survey of compliance with a ventilator care bundle following the
introduction of a clinical information system in a cardiac intensive
care unit, *ACTA Blackpool* 2009.

Box 9.8

Research evidence

Computerized guideline for glucose regulation has been shown to
improve glucose control in intensive care.

E. Rood, R. J. Bosman, J. I. van der Spoel, P. Taylor and D. F. Zandstra,
2005. Use of a computerized guideline for glucose regulation in the
intensive care unit improved both guideline adherence and glucose
regulation, *Journal of the American Medical Informatics Association*
12(2): 172–80.

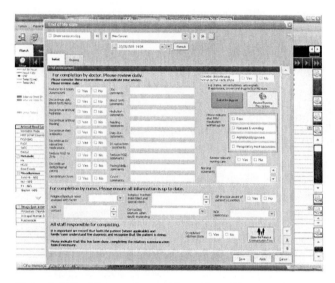

Figure 9.4 Checklists can be used to guide and improve care.

Checklists

Checklists for procedures are becoming standard in critical care medicine as a way to manage complex patient care (Figure 9.4).

A CIS, particularly if it is user-customizable, can support the writing and changing of checklists.

It is easy to insert them into the workflow at the appropriate place. There are almost endless possibilities for the areas where checklists can be used, for example preparation for transfer, intravascular catheter care, tracheostomy decannulation.

As a unit becomes familiar and comfortable with a CIS, more checklists can be added. It is important that the number of checklists is not allowed to proliferate unduly as this can slow workflow and lead to resentment.

Handover

Handover can often be affected by introduction of a CIS, especially if all paper documents are dispensed with.

Studies of handovers illustrate that handover is often about gathering data from many sources to give a total picture to the healthcare professional coming on duty. It is a time when healthcare professionals take personal notes to support their memory of the tasks they need to do and the important issues.

A CIS that requires handovers to be carried out entirely within the formalized structure may not allow individuals to organize information in the way that works best for them, reducing the effectiveness of recall.

While improving handover and reducing inefficiencies is worthwhile, it is important not to take away the informal tools that people use to do their jobs, as this may create resentment and reduce the quality of work.

Box 9.9
Research evidence
Handover is a complex human interaction that requires multiple skills and uses multiple supports.

C. Tang and S. Carpendale, 2007. An observational study on information flow during nurses' shift change. In *Proceedings of the*

SIGCHI Conference on Human Factors in Computing Systems. San José, CA: ACM, pp. 219–28.

Multi-professional teamwork

The introduction of a CIS is likely to affect the work of all members of the multi-professional team.

It may impact team members such as dieticians and pharmacists, who may not be permanently based in the critical care unit. For example, facilities such as remote access to the CIS from other locations in a hospital may enable informed consultation with allied health professionals, without requiring a visit to the unit.

For dieticians, integration of dietetic protocols and records in the CIS will increase their accessibility for unit staff. It is unlikely that this will lead to improved patient nutrition unless work practices are changed to take advantage of them.

Box 9.10
Research evidence

The introduction of a CIS with a link to the feed protocol in a cardiothoracic CCU was not found to improve the adequacy of nutritional support. The combination of a visual display of energy balance, a feeding protocol, and an adequate prescribing method for feed were identified as necessary to achieve improvements in patients' nutritional intake.

Remote access may be significant for pharmacists, allowing them to check patients' medications while working in the pharmacy.

There are a number of other ways in which a CIS may affect their work. The improved, electronic documentation that a CIS provides can assist pharmacy stock control, for example. Accurate estimates of drug usage can be obtained from the CIS as it can compute what has been used across patients and the enforced use of scientific names (as opposed to brand names) makes accounting easier.

A CIS linked to the pharmacy system can stop the ordering of drugs that are unavailable, saving time for both clinicians and pharmacists by looking for alternatives immediately.

Ward rounds

Given the significance of ward rounds to multidisciplinary teamworking, they may be particularly sensitive to changes associated with the introduction of a CIS.

Compared with paper records, the computer screen may be visible to only a few team members at one time, the data displayed will be controlled by one person at a time (giving rise to a 'fight for the mouse'), as will data entry. Other team members may therefore be excluded from discussion of the patient, and may lose interest in the ward round, unless deliberate efforts are made to involve them.

The introduction of a CIS can affect the status hierarchy in a ward-round team as junior staff are typically more computer literate than senior staff and may acquire a more central, and potentially influential, role in retrieving and entering data. Senior staff may respond by treating juniors as secretaries who do their keyboard work for them, or seek to retain control by using the CIS themselves.

The introduction of a CIS can therefore lead to different ward rounds having quite distinct characters depending on who is leading.

Influences include how comfortable the lead clinician is with the CIS, the extent to which they consider it helpful to have access to large amounts of up-to-date data for their decision-making, and their attention to team dynamics.

Different ward rounds might therefore involve only a few doctors in discussion of large volumes of data retrieved from the CIS, the senior doctor may stand back from use of the CIS, leaving that to juniors, or the ward-round leader might make efforts to engage all team members in discussion by arranging the group around the CIS screen so that everyone can see and inviting them to suggest what data should be displayed.

Box 9.11

Research evidence

Morrison *et al.* describe how multidisciplinary interaction during the ward can be decreased, depending on the ergonomic set-up of the CIS. For bedside reviews, they observe that if the consultant is logged into the CIS during the discussion, it can be helpful for them to stand slightly further back from the screen so that they can see everyone and ensure that they log-out before the end of the discussion to encourage interaction.

C. Morrison, M. Jones, A. Blackwell and A. Vuylsteke, 2008. Electronic patient record use during ward rounds: a qualitative study of interaction between medical staff, *Critical Care* 12(6): R148.

Changes to the workflow

The previous section has listed many of the benefits of having a CIS. To achieve these benefits, work practices, and often the workflow, change. This section puts forward some of the changes in workflow that may be expected and discusses how to maximize the benefit by addressing possible problems.

Disrupting the workflow

Disruption of workflow is one of the main reasons cited for failure of a CIS. A poor match between workflow and CIS design can occur for a number of reasons.

It could be that the CIS was poorly designed, or designed for a different medical system and transported across borders. Such an issue can be resolved through careful choice of CIS or through a customizable CIS, particularly one that is user-customizable. In the latter case, workflows can be adjusted as necessary as they change and develop.

Poor alignment of a CIS to the workflow can occur if there is not significant user involvement in the selection and customization of the CIS. If CIS design is undertaken primarily by non-users, assumptions about how the workflow ought to be may differ from how things are done, with the result that the CIS does not match local work practices. It is possible to idealize, and over-formalize, the way that practices work to communicate to IT professionals, with a similar problematic outcome.

Another common issue that affects the design of the workflow is the negotiation of different disciplines' and departments' needs. If clinicians and management, or clinicians across departments, have dissimilar needs, this can lead to conflict, non-use and hospital rejection of the system.

A CIS that matches clinical workflow is essential, and is a common factor among systems that are successfully implemented. Systems customizable by their users are particularly useful for creating a workflow. Such systems support the development and changing of workflow over time, something likely to occur when the CIS becomes embedded in the way the unit works.

Box 9.12
Research evidence

Han *et al.* point to a number of disruptions to their workflow that lead to an unexpected increase in mortality.

Y. Y. Han, J. A. Carcillo, S. T. Venkataraman *et al.*, 2005. Unexpected increased mortality after implementation of a commercially sold computerized physician order entry system, *Pediatrics* 116(6): 1506–12.

User involvement increases the likelihood that a system will match the workflow, but Bossen describes how clinicians can over-formalize their work when describing it.

C. Bossen, 2006. Representations at work: a national standard for electronic patient records. In *Proceedings of the Conference on Computer Supported Cooperative Work*, Banff, Alberta, Canada, pp. 69–78.

Scott *et al.* describe how conflicts in data needs between clinicians and managers can lead to the avoidance, and ultimate failure, of a system. Martin *et al.* describe the difficulties of managing different needs across multiple units in an institution. They give an example that in an emergency department nurses were required to click through nine screens to enter one piece of essential data because the data were not used elsewhere in the hospital.

J. Scott, T. Rundall, T. Vogt and J. Hsu, 2005. Kaiser Permanente's experience of implementing an electronic patient record: a qualitative study, *British Medical Journal* 331: 1313–16.

D. Martin, M. Rouncefield, J. O'Neill, M. Hartswood and D. Randall, 2005. Timing in the art of integration: 'that's how the Bastille got stormed'. In *Proceedings of the 2005 International ACM SIGGROUP Conference on Supporting Group Work*, Association for Computing Machinery. Available at: http://portal.acm.org/citation.cfm?id=1099256.

Time saving

Time saving is often expected to be a benefit of CIS use, but experience suggests that this is rarely realized.

Some aspects of using the CIS are slower. Reviewing data across multiple screens, for example, takes greater effort and time. Searching in the history becomes feasible with the CIS, but takes time. Other mundane parts of using CIS, such as logging in, waiting for data to load or the screen to refresh, and the keyboard entry of data, can offset any time savings.

In particular, ward rounds sometimes become longer. This is certainly true while clinicians are initially learning to use the system, but in addition the greater range of data means that there is more to make sense of and discuss. With one point of access to the record at a particular location, some activities, such as checking drug prescriptions, that could previously have been done in parallel now also have to be done in series.

Integration with rest of hospital

Integrating with the rest of the hospital or other relevant parties, such as general practitioners, can be a challenge if they do not have the same system.

Given the diversity of clinical systems available, this will often be the case (unless there is some central authority, probably related to funding, that can enforce standardization).

Care will therefore be necessary in planning the transfer of information between units before the CIS is implemented. This will need to address matters such as which data items need to be shared, in what format, how they will be shared and with what frequency and response times.

Without suitable interfaces between systems it may be necessary to print out a summary of the CIS record. It is not always easy to do this in a format and at a level of detail that will meet the requirements of all parties with whom data needs to be shared. CIS use may lead to an increase in paper use where a hardcopy of the CIS record needs to be made.

Paper saving

It is widely believed that the introduction of a CIS will eliminate paper usage on the ward. This is generally not the case.

Paper use is likely to continue, and sometimes even increase, with the introduction of a CIS.

Box 9.13
Research evidence

An analysis of the persistence of paper use following the introduction of a fully integrated CIS in a large centre identified 11 reasons why clinical staff retained paper, including efficiency (in terms of established work processes), ease of use, task specificity, customized data layout, trust and security. For example, a number of clinicians prepared personal notes on the treatment plans for particular patients and found that the personalization, portability and speed of access of paper made it more helpful than the CIS.

J. J. Saleem, A. L. Russ, C. F. Justice *et al.*, 2009. Exploring the persistence of paper with the electronic health record. *International Journal of Medical Informatics* 78(9): 618–28.

The persistence of paper may be a potential source of medical errors, where paper-based ward rounds are used to circumvent CIS processes, or where data recorded on paper are not subsequently entered in the CIS, creating gaps in the record. While efforts to eliminate paper use altogether risk being counter-productive, because of the advantages that paper offers in some respects, it is nevertheless important to ensure that paper use is integrated with the CIS and does not undermine it. For example, allowing staff to print out personalized patient lists from the CIS may encourage greater integration than forbidding such printouts and having staff develop their own informal lists.

Paper remains as a way to integrate with other systems. For example, wards that do not use a CIS will require paper copies of charts.

It may be necessary to produce a paper version of the CIS record if there is a system failure at any time. Such situations may be the cause of increased paper usage as CIS output is often not designed to optimize paper usage and may generate large amounts of paper with a low information density.

Communication

A CIS is likely to change patterns of communication between staff (Figure 9.5). The ability to work remotely decreases ad-hoc communication that happens when staff bump into each other on the unit and at the bedside. This can lead to less communication and less of a sense of team interaction. It can lead to more formal communication, which leaves out some important details that may be too sensitive for the notes, such as emotional state.

On the other hand a CIS may mean less interruption from constant communication and may increase efficiency.

The evidence is not definitive either way, so it is important to monitor for possible negative consequences.

Patients

While a CIS can free up staff time in some situations, enabling them to interact more with patients, it can distract staff attention from patients.

October 2006   February 2007

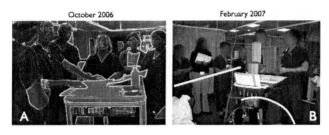

November 2007

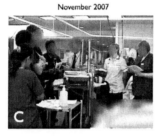

Figure 9.5 Introduction of a CIS will impact on communication. These pictures show (A) the team dynamic around chart tables, (B) CIS with the team excluded from discussion and eventually (C) discussion around the CIS.

The large amount of data presented can be overwhelming and entice the clinician to focus on the data rather than examining or interacting directly with the patient.

Although there is no research to say that such situations lead to better or worse patient care, patients have mentioned that it is disconcerting to be ignored. In one centre, initial feedback from patients following implementation of the CIS was that the nurses spent all their time playing computer games!

A CIS may encourage the use of 'sitting ward rounds' where the clinical team (or a subset of it) meet in a room away from the patients, with the CIS projected on a wall, or allow remote working, reducing the visibility of clinicians to patients and the opportunities for interaction.

Finally, the excitement, and sometimes anxiety, around interacting with a new CIS can mean that many staff may congregate around the computer at the end of a patient's bed. The resultant noise and lack of focus on the patient's needs can be a negative experience for patients.

Mobile devices

The need to have accurate patient information and reference material at the bedside has prompted research into the use of mobile devices in critical care.

One study found that clinicians thought of the devices as convenient and functional, but equivalent to paper. The study concluded that handheld computers have potential in the CCU, but the information accessed needs to be integrated and the system developed specifically for the critical care environment.

Box 9.14
Research evidence
A systematic review of 13 studies of the use of personal digital assistants (PDAs) identified that handheld devices had a positive effect in areas of rapid response, error prevention and data management and accessibility. Insufficient evidence was available, however, to say whether these devices improved outcomes and workflow efficiencies because of their mobility.

M. Prgomet, A. Georgiou and J. I. Westbrook, 2009. The impact of mobile handheld technology on hospital physicians' work practices and patient care: a systematic review. *Journal of the American Medical Informatics Association* 16(6): 792–801.

S. E. Lapinsky, J. Weshler, S. Mehta *et al.*, 2001. Handheld computers in critical care, *Critical Care* 5: 227–31.

As many critical care units have a computer at each bedside, mobile devices may be more useful during interactions such as the ward round. Mobile devices are still developing, so their use in the future may change, but it would seem likely that speed of data entry and visibility of screens by more than one person at a time may constrain their use in critical care.

Key point

- The beneficial influence of the CIS on workflows is achieved through careful attention to details.

TO LEARN MORE

A. J. Sellen and R. H. R. Harper, 2003. *The Myth of the Paperless Office*, 2nd edn. Cambridge, MA: MIT Press.

Chapter 10

Research and audit

Introduction

A CIS can open new possibilities to utilize data for research and audit.

When set up appropriately for data extraction, a query that may have taken a day of clinical time when records were held on paper can now be done in a matter of minutes, or even seconds.

This chapter discusses the ways that available data in a CIS can be utilized and examines the problems that such a large database might present and strategies to handle them.

Data for research and audit

Very large amounts of data are collected in the CIS database.

Fortunately, data files are usually small, after a number of years amounting to gigabytes rather than terabytes – usually equivalent in size to a high definition DVD and easily stored on an external hard drive.

Therefore the CIS database presents a considerable opportunity for research, whether specified research projects or just personal queries to support clinical development.

Audit and benchmarking are more easily done.

A CIS can be set up to collate data needed to comply with national standards, provide data on the incidence of 'errors', or to retrieve data for a coroner's inquest.

The CIS ensures that the data are all in one place, that records are not missing and that they are legible. Their digital form makes them searchable for quicker use, allows data to be digitally copied, avoiding transcription errors, and in some cases data can be automatically extracted to templates for easy scanning.

The CIS makes actions taken traceable to a specific person, a useful feature when a problem or unusual circumstance arises.

In addition to making data easier to obtain for current standard requests, a CIS allows for more complicated audits for the development of the institution. For example, the CIS can track compliance with protocols, resource usage, or other institution-specific benchmarking that management or senior clinicians may find useful.

Doing research and audit with a CIS database

Extracting the data

The ability to extract data from the CIS database is crucial to using the database.

When deciding which CIS to purchase, vendors should be asked about how data can be extracted from the CIS. To be useful for research, the data must be in a raw format, such as an xml or other database file.

Data in more familiar formats, such as a pdf file, may look nice but will be difficult to extract and use for a range of research queries.

It is best to look for systems in which data can be exported into formats that can be read by common software, such as Excel or Access.

Next consider whether the data are in a form that can be computed, or whether the data need to be manipulated. For example, if a research project needs data on three parameters for each patient, and the data export to Excel in just one column (rather than three) it will be necessary to use some programming techniques, such as pivot tables, to put the data in an appropriate form.

It is best to avoid data that will require complex manipulation before it can be used as this introduces a potential source of error.

The final step in testing the feasibility of data extraction is to try to extract some data. If this proves difficult or requires specialist knowledge of the structure of the database or programming tools, it will be necessary to establish whether the resources to do this are likely to be available in everyday use, or the database will risk becoming a 'roach motel' where data get trapped inside, but cannot get out.

Using the data

To be useful for research and audit, data need to be categorized in such a way that they can be easily interrogated.

One reason this is difficult is that computers use mathematical logic to select data, requiring clinicians to think differently about patients than they might usually do in their clinical work. For example, it may not be possible to extract all patients with condition X, but most of these patients may be identifiable using proxies, such as patients with a heart rate greater than 180 beats/minute. If such difficulties can be overcome, the CIS can be a fantastic resource for research.

The problem is typically that of too much data, such that it can lead to 'drunk and lamppost' research that forms the research questions around the data, rather than collecting the data needed to answer the research question. Establishing a clear clinical premise, before considering how the CIS can provide the data, should help to avoid this problem.

A bigger problem is who the data are for and therefore, what data are collected. Research and managerial audit requests usually query the data in different ways and would therefore prefer the database structured in sometimes conflicting ways. Moreover, the CIS should be primarily a tool for caring for patients, which may require the data to be structured in a third way, creating a tension about which data should be collected.

The opportunity that a CIS provides to access data at a fine level of detail often attracts the interest of staff, such as managers and researchers, who may seek to require clinicians to collect additional data for their needs. Clinical staff are likely to resent filling in many data fields unrelated to the clinical process, as this is time-consuming and draws them away from caring for patients. It is important to consider closely which data are needed and the effects on staff of collecting them.

Ensuring data quality

The quality of research or audit depends on the quality of the data in the system – as the saying goes: garbage in, garbage out.

People using a CIS may not always be careful about filling in fields that are not relevant to them; this can happen with paper documentation. One way to deal with this is to have fields automatically filled in, or made part of a checklist.

Studies of CIS use suggest that clinical staff can sometimes validate numbers way out of range or tick off everything on a checklist without reading it. Using the facility of showing 'last valued entered' in a field when a form is opened is attractive as in theory it means staff only have to re-enter data when there has been a change – however, experience has shown that this information is often not rechecked, meaning out-of-date data can be validated. Those using the CIS for research should therefore inspect the data carefully to make sure it is not full of outliers and wherever possible use some other form of triangulation to check the data.

In some CIS systems, especially user-customizable ones, it may be possible to encourage good data entry by not allowing forms to be submitted, or data to be validated, that are not in the appropriate range. While this tactic may work for a while, staff may be discouraged from using the CIS if the burden this imposes proves onerous and may devise work-arounds (entering the minimum data needed to 'satisfy' the CIS even if this is not clinically appropriate) to allow them, as they see it, to get on with their job.

For example, clinicians may enter a generic diagnosis as this brings up a shorter checklist, even though they are aware that the patient has a specific condition.

To improve the quality of data it is therefore necessary to find ways for the clinical staff to benefit from high-quality data – either through being the direct recipients of research or incorporating the data collection measures into the appropriate part of the care process so that it helps them care. People are more likely to enter high-quality data if they see the benefits of doing so.

Understanding your data

The CIS offers a vast resource for investigating what is happening in a unit. For example, it can identify how many patients have received the most expensive drug in a year or how many care bundles are completed on average. Having easy access to such data can lead to a focus primarily on what is happening in the unit. Fixing a problem in the unit, though, requires an understanding of why it is happening.

It is important to move beyond easy access to data, seeing it only as the first step to exploration that can solve the problem.

Box 10.1

A critial care unit noticed that only 93% of care bundles were being completed by the nursing staff. If the enquiry had stopped here, the clinical management might have started to pressure nurses to complete more care bundles. After looking into why they were not completed, however, it turned out that the bundles that were not being completed were ones that required clinical intervention and were therefore not in the nurses' control.

Resourcing data mining

Once the database of the CIS becomes relatively populated, many people will want access to the data for research and audit. Managers might want a report about bed days, or a researcher might want data about a specific action in specific patients. Responding to these requests will require someone familiar with the data structure and the extraction tools, who is unlikely to be the person who requested the data.

Key points

- A CIS provides large quantities of data that can be used for research audit.
- Issues may arise when using this data including how they are extracted and how they can be extracted regularly in high volumes.
- If these issues are addressed, the CIS will give benefits to many and can be an important factor in convincing people of its success.

Chapter 11

CIS of the future

Lessons learned

This section gathers together some of the key points about CIS that have been discussed throughout the book.

CIS does not have to be a disaster

Contrary to widespread belief, the introduction of a CIS can be extremely productive for an institution, but it takes a lot of hard work and attention.

Effort must be put into choosing the right system for the institution and considerable work must be done to prepare both individuals and the institution for change.

Despite fears about CIS, most people adapt to it quickly and easily

The idea of CIS often causes anxiety and fear for clinical staff, but once it has arrived, staff usually adapt and find it useful.

As discussed in Chapters 2 and 3, fear can be addressed by involving people in the preparation and selection processes. If staff can be coaxed to use it for a year, it is very unlikely that they will want to return to paper.

New staff joining an institution will quickly learn the system, accepting it as a natural part of a unit.

Buying a CIS is part of an ongoing process

Buying the CIS is only the first step in a long journey of integrating the CIS into an institution and its clinical practice. Once staff realize what it can do for their work, there will be continued demand for improvements.

In addition to the energy and costs of improving the system, it will also need to be maintained with regular hardware and software upgrades. As mentioned in Chapter 2, the system is likely to cost five to eight times the initial cost over its lifetime.

A CIS can only be as good as the organization allows

A well-designed CIS will not work if the organizational culture and structure do not support it. A CIS cannot be used to force change in an institution's work culture. Changes must precede the CIS and then be supported by it. This lesson underscores the importance of involving as many users as possible in the selection of the CIS.

Clinical leadership is essential to the success of a CIS

Clinical buy-in and leadership are crucial components in the selection and implementation of a CIS. Such leadership requires more than just lip service; it requires active participation in the selection of the CIS, in the preparation of the institution for its arrival and in the use of the system once implemented.

A CIS provides new ways of looking at patients

One of the greatest benefits of a CIS is the opportunity to look at patients in new ways. More kinds of data are available and they can be combined in new ways. This is particularly true in user-customizable systems in which the users have control over which data are collected and how they are displayed. This can ensure that the system provides the data that users want rather than those the system developers believe the users want (or those that are the easiest for them to provide given the way the system is designed).

A CIS is unlikely to save time

It is often claimed that a CIS will save clinical staff time, but it is well known that work expands to fill the time available. Although some tasks will be quicker, others will be slower.

Benefits of the system are more likely to come from new, safer, and more productive ways of working rather than efficiency-savings.

The national picture

Many countries are promoting the use of electronic patient records and clinical information systems. These are seen to improve patient safety, to increase the portability of patient records, and to be a useful mechanism to gather aggregated data for healthcare policy planning. These reasons for establishing a nationwide clinical information system may not be entirely the same as those an institution would have for putting them in and may lead to conflicts about which system is appropriate. It is useful to understand the relevant national approach and the reasons for it. In this section the two extreme end-points for national (or institutional) strategies, centralized and decentralized, are explained.

Centralized approach

A centralized approach is an attempt to create a single standard system for a whole country or institution and is usually driven from the top down.

This was the approach adopted in the UK's National Programme for Information Technology that, initially at least, sought to pursue a policy of 'ruthless standardization'. It has the advantages of significant economies of scale, ensured interoperability and central control over important issues such as security, reliability and consistency.

Such monolithic systems are inflexible and are rarely suitable for all institutions (or, if employed within an institution, for all units/departments). They prevent local initiative and innovation, which have been an important part of the advance of technology use in medicine. These systems are slow to develop, as they require the whole system to work at once and contain significant additional costs (not to mention possible local distress) of replacing legacy systems.

Decentralized approach

The alternative decentralized approach focuses on data interchange standards that all systems on the market must comply with. This approach allows independent applications and systems to communicate easily with each other, without defining how they are organized internally. The open nature of the standard makes it difficult for vendors, particularly large ones, to lock institutions into a particular system because proprietary data standards will not be supported.

Developing a national system in this way is bottom up and relies on local initiative, thereby ensuring that solutions are adapted to local conditions. This is the approach adopted in the USA, reflecting the existence of multiple powerful players in the healthcare marketplace (e.g. health maintenance organizations, insurance companies) who can resist any centralized system.

The complexity of clinical information systems and their constant evolution means that open data standards may not cover everything and interoperability between applications or systems could be limited. The range of choices available on the market, and the implementation process being left up to each institution, could mean that there is variability in the success of utilizing clinical information systems and that there may be sub-optimal solutions.

A mix of both

There may be solutions between the two extremes. For example, a customizable system, particularly if customization is done by the users, can build in both interoperability as well as flexibility, treading the middle ground.

In countries with centralized national strategies, individual units will need to raise questions about its customizability and consider what preparation work will need to be done to ensure its success within the work patterns and culture of their institution. If the approach is more decentralized then there will be more room for choice, and decisions on many of the issues discussed in this book will need to be taken at a unit level.

Critical care is a specialized area which may not be specifically addressed in a national strategy. Nevertheless, the national approach is still likely to influence local CIS implementation to some degree, if only in setting data standards, so attention will need to be paid to it.

CIS of the future

The structure of the CIS of the future will depend upon which approach is taken nationally.

It may be a proprietary, seamless, integrated system or one made from open, interoperable and substitutable components. In all cases, it will have a number of implications for the way that medicine is practised.

Working across boundaries

Medicine traditionally has strong boundaries between disciplines and institutions, despite repeated research findings that have shown that multidisciplinary teams, particularly in complex areas of healthcare such as critical care, are more effective in providing care. It is well known that many mistakes in care occur when a patient crosses institutional boundaries. Patient care can be dramatically improved by working across boundaries to achieve better integration.

This problem is in part practical, with the need for better communication infrastructures, as well as a cultural one of change. The future CIS will facilitate greater multidisciplinary working and will allow, and perhaps require, the crossing of intra- and inter-organization boundaries. Although it cannot solve the cultural issues of crossing boundaries it can go a long way to solving practical communication issues to smooth the way.

Mobile working

Healthcare has traditionally been provided in primary care centres, such as GP offices, or in large secondary care institutions, such as hospitals, as these places provided the necessary infrastructure, such as patient records and reference material. The advent of mobile computing now means that healthcare records and reference material can potentially be accessed from anywhere, changing the possibilities of where healthcare is provided.

In hospital, more work can now be done at the bedside as useful data are always to hand. Mobile computing could also change the location of healthcare altogether, which could now take place in the community, in a patient's home, or through a remote telecare situation such as video conferencing. There may also be situations in the future when healthcare is not done synchronously, meaning that the patient and clinician do not interact at the same time, but rather at different times through email or text.

Personalized healthcare

There is a general medical trend towards the personalization of healthcare. This is a result, in part, of advances in genetics, but also of the greater amount of data that can be queried to show similar cases. Technology is opening up new possibilities for personalized healthcare. New technologies are supporting patients in the self-care of long-term conditions under the supervision of clinical staff. For example, a patient with chronic obstructive pulmonary disorder may be on a specific diet, the maintenance of which is supported by interactive technology, and their progress is checked weekly by a dietician through the data sent by the device back to the CIS. Other examples are access by a patient to his or her health record.

Data-driven healthcare

CIS provides a wealth of data that can be explored to improve care, whether through more active use of data on a case-by-case basis or through research. CIS also offers the possibility of clinical decision support. This is sometimes wrongly perceived as the computer making choices rather than the clinician, but this is not the case. Clinical decision support can range from juxtaposing critical data on a graph, to checks on drug interactions or allergies, to some systems which propose actions based on rules drawn from medical textbooks (but clinicians must decide whether to follow these actions or not).

Currently, most clinical decision support is of the first two types, as the latter faces a number of organizational and technical problems. Clinicians do not like being told what to do and often find the lack of subtlety in current clinical decision support systems frustrating. New designs are finding ways to determine possible useful data and present it at decision-making points. For example, a system described by Bates *et al.* (2003) provides the most recent serum potassium level when digoxin is being ordered. This allows the physician to use this potentially helpful information if they choose.

One interesting development in this area is clinical decision support based on a particular patient's data. Most intensive care monitoring systems are based on population data and do not take into account the variability among individual patients' characteristics. Research into patient-specific alarm algorithms that work in real time is now being done.

Key points

- National electronic patient records programmes may not address critical care directly, but are likely to set standards that local CISs will need to adhere to.

- The CIS of the future will facilitate multidisciplinary working across traditional intra- and inter-organizational boundaries and will need to support the delivery of more geographically dispersed and personalized healthcare.
- CISs provide a wealth of data that offers the potential for more data-driven healthcare, but the data need to be presented in ways that support rather than override clinical decision-making.

TO LEARN MORE

D. W. Bates, G. J. Kuperman, S. Wang *et al.*, 2003. Ten commandments for effective clinical decision support: making the practice of evidence-based medicine a reality, *Journal of the American Medical Informatics Association* 10: 523–30.

Y. Zhang and P. Szolovits, 2008. Patient-specific learning in real time for adaptive monitoring in critical care, *Journal of Biomedical Informatics* 41(3): 452–60.

INDEX